RELATIVE
MATTERS

RELATIVE MATTERS

The essential guide to finding your way
around the care system for older people

CHRIS MOON-WILLEMS

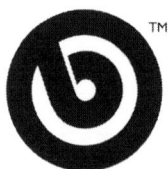

bookshaker

First Published in Great Britain 2012
by www.BookShaker.com

FULLY REVISED AND UPDATED 2014

I dedicate this book to my parents
who have taught me so much
and made me the person I am proud of today.

ACKNOWLEDGEMENTS

I would like to begin by thanking all the older people and their relatives, whom I have had the pleasure of working with over the years for teaching me so much. Their unique stories have often been humbling and full of rich and inspirational content. What a generation!

A big thank you to Doctor Simon Duffy, a well known social innovator and writer, whose innovative and inspirational approach paved the way for personal budgets. Simon influenced my practice significantly and ignited my passion for designing services around the individual, rather than making the person fit off-the-shelf services. He is a true visionary and master of change.

I would also like to thank my business mentor Richard White, for his support and encouragement to write this book and for helping me take my business to the next level.

Thank you also to Louise Wilby for her patience, advice and diligent pursuit of technical accuracy.

I also thank the fine operation at *Bookshaker* for the gift of Lucy McCarraher, my editor. She has been a supporter and tolerant editor from day one and her magic and skill has helped me craft this book.

I would also like to thank my sons, Matt and Simon, along with Roger, Lindsay and Bryan, my brother, sister and brother-in-law, for their encouragement in writing this book and for their generous love and support while I was writing it.

Finally I would like to thank my parents. They have taught me more than any book or training course about the challenges of growing older and being "on the other side" of the care system. Indeed, this book would not exist without them, neither would I have ever experienced the privilege of supporting two people I love and care about on their final journey. I will be forever grateful for the valuable insights they have given me.

CONTENTS

Acknowledgements

Contents

Foreword

FOREWORD

One of the perks about being asked to write a foreword is that one gets to read the book first. Having worked with someone professionally for many years and being aware of the extent of a talent that, in spite of extensive experience in public service, had only been partially realised, I read through this book with increasing admiration for what Chris Moon-Willems has achieved. There has never been a more important time for this authoritative and unique publication. Almost daily we are made painfully aware of the economic and social consequences relating to our increasingly elderly and dependent population. Health and Social Care managers, of which I was one for forty years, have become increasingly challenged by the rapidly rising numbers of people needing help and the dwindling availability of funds to support them. Successive governments have attempted to re-organise structures and introduce policies that will improve provisions for and enhance the lives of older people while at the same time reducing overall costs. From Care Management, changes to social security funding of residential care, tighter eligibility criteria, and increasingly complex welfare benefits, successive governments have grappled with the problem of cost-control while meeting need and maintaining quality. Running through all the reforms has been the theme of individualisation or personalisation, the provision of services to meet the needs of the individual, about which the author has long been an ardent advocate. With the best of intentions, however, what has been created is a maze of bureaucratic complexity, which can defeat even the most determined of those seeking to understand "the system". In writing this book Chris draws on her unparalleled experience as a local authority practitioner and manager to guide us through the maze, utilising the knowledge she gained when working on the project to personalise health and social care budgets. It is a book about practice; written from the heart, and littered liberally with gems of insight and practical tips. It will be invaluable to anyone who needs information about how best to support their elderly and dependent friends and relatives. It is both highly personal and supremely professional. The insights are full of warmth and enormously moving. They will give heart to those struggling, as Chris has, with their feelings about their parents becoming elderly and dependent and how feelings can sometimes get in the way of knowing what to do for the best. This is an easy book to read and find one's way around; but readers should not be deceived by its simplicity. It has profoundly important messages not only for individuals but also for professionals at every level involved in the business of planning and providing care and services for older people. It provides a wealth of meticulously referenced useful information. The stories are all anonymised illustrations from practice, which provide authenticity and authority. The subject-focused reference section at the end will be invaluable for further help and signposting. The *Points to Remember* sections add further authenticity and personalisation to a text that is always relevant and immediate. This is an invaluable book for anyone involved in planning care for elderly loved ones.

Margaret Bamford, OBE.
Deputy Lord Lieutenant
CEO Leaves of Hope Charity for children in Belarus

INTRODUCTION

"Brenda Mason!" the nurse called out in the A & E department at our local hospital. Mum had fallen again and this time she had cut open her head. We had been at the hospital for more than three hours and this was our eighth visit in the past year. I kept looking at my watch, as I had to get back to work but didn't want to leave her.

I have worked with older people for most of my working life, in the NHS and during my long career in Social Services. I was a nursing assistant in a geriatric hospital and supported people in the community. I have managed residential care homes; home care services, hospital discharge and day services. I also specialised in care of the elderly during my professional training. However, nothing taught me as much as caring for my elderly parents, or prepared me for the emotional turmoil I would go through as their health deteriorated and dependency increased.

My parents have been happily married for more than sixty years and worked hard before they retired. My mother worked as a secretary and my father as clerk of works for a major airline. I was the eldest of three children and have a younger brother and sister. We enjoyed camping holidays abroad when we were growing up, which was not so common in those days. My parents loved to travel and enjoyed visiting friends and family in Australia as well as travelling to other countries across the globe.

My mother, who is eighty-five years-old, has been troubled with poor health for most of her adult life, spending long periods in hospital for kidney and back problems and undergoing electric shock treatment for depression when I was growing up. She has a number of chronic health conditions, has been challenged by a poor memory for more than twenty years and suffers from severe anxiety and depression.

My father, who is nearly ninety years old and is registered as a blind person, has been the primary carer for my mother for many years. Now his own health and memory have deteriorated to the point where we need to consider other options for Mum's care and support.

I noticed little clues that led me to this conclusion: piles of bills and correspondence lying around, food in the fridge past its "use by" date, weeds in the garden and the lawn needing a good cut. Conversation with them focused on the challenges they were facing, their health and continence issues.

Dad had become forgetful and was looking more tired than usual. Mum was sleeping more during the day and bothering less with her appearance.

Both my parents have become increasingly dependent over the past few years and regularly get frustrated. I have also struggled with their loss of independence. Instead of going to my parents for advice, I have needed to put my worries aside as they increasingly rely on me to overcome the problems they are facing. We have reversed positions. They need me and just as they were always there for me, I have chosen to be there for them.

You may be recognising that your mother, father or elderly aunt is slowing down and finding it difficult to get in and out of the bath. Maybe they keep losing things or you notice that the food in their fridge is past its "use by" date.

In my experience, the transition to older people needing support services or moving into a care or nursing home does not happen gradually or as the result of careful planning. It usually follows a sudden change or deterioration in their health. Some of the events that can trigger these changes are:

- Death of their spouse or partner.
- A sudden illness such as a stroke or heart attack.

- Deteriorating health generally, lethargy, avoidance of going out claiming they tire easily.
- Disinterest in hobbies and going out with friends.
- Diagnosis of cancer, Parkinson's Disease or other degenerative illness.
- An accident, for example a fall resulting in a fractured femur with associated loss of confidence.
- Deterioration in memory and the ability to process information or sequence tasks.

Looking after elderly relatives can be a satisfying though difficult experience. For example we may feel that, because we love our parents, we want to help as they become frailer and less able to do things for themselves. At this stage of their lives, it is our last chance to show our love and to help them as they once helped us when we were children. This reversal of child and parent roles isn't always easy. However much we love our parents there will often be a tension between wanting to do our best for them and wanting to live our own life. It is quite normal to feel like this, so don't worry about it.

Talking with family, friends and colleagues I became aware that there are many people looking after or worried about an elderly relative, typically their parents. This is not surprising when we consider that life expectancy is increasing and people are living longer, although not necessarily in good health. Indeed we are on the brink of a population explosion and will see a dramatic rise in the number of people over eighty-five years of age in the years ahead.

People are also putting off having a family until later, resulting in an increasing number of men and women who are beginning to worry about their ageing parents at the same time as looking after their growing family. This is why we are often referred to as the sandwich generation. The trend for women to stay at home to look after our children has also changed. Many now return to work after having a child due to financial necessity or because they want to continue their career. Torn between the demands of caring for our adult children and sometimes grandchildren, our career and ageing parents can leave us feeling overwhelmed, emotionally drained and resentful. The situation becomes even worse if we live a long way from our parents.

Brothers, sisters and in-laws each have their own perception of how much time and responsibility should be given to supporting parents and will have varying amounts of baggage from their parent-child relationship. This, as well as the distance that family members live apart and other commitments, may mean that caring for elderly parents often falls on one person's shoulders, more often a daughter's. If you are single, like me, you also lack a partner to share the fears, frustrations and celebrations of caring for your parents on a day-to-day basis.

We all have different ways of showing our parents that we love them and there is no right or wrong way to do it. For me it is not how much time we spend with our parents, it is the quality of the time we spend with them and our willingness to look beyond their words, with determination to help them resolve whatever difficulties they are facing.

Notwithstanding the challenges of sharing my parents' last journey with them, I wouldn't miss it for anything and I invite you to join me so that, together, we can learn lessons from the experience. I will also reflect on my professional experience of working with older people and help you to understand the resources available in plain language rather than medical or social work jargon.

I have written this book with two observations in mind. Firstly, the increasing number of people I know who are worried about, or struggling with caring for elderly parents or other relatives. Secondly, most elderly people have to fund their own care and find it difficult to navigate the complex care system without a social worker to support them. People who don't qualify for support from Social Services are often left to find their own way in a bewildering environment where they have little idea about where to begin.

The care system is complex and confusing. As a result there are a wealth of different options to choose from and possible pathways to take. Older people and their relatives often need considerable assistance to navigate the system. By the time they gain access to the right information and advice for their particular circumstances, they have often made a lot of wrong turns and wasted time and money.

Many of us have a good understanding of the needs of our elderly relatives and the difficulties they are facing, but much less idea of what solutions are available and how we might gain access to them. It is not only broad information and advice about what support is available that we need, but an assessment of our own situation and consideration of all the available options. In practice, we are rarely experts in social care or the NHS and have poor information on which to base our decisions.

It is for these reasons that I set up an elderly care consultancy, also called Relative Matters, www.relativematters.org which provides independent advice, and practical, skilled and experienced help for relatives to help them choose, find and arrange care solutions for their elderly loved ones. This might be care in someone's home, a residential or nursing home, respite care, equipment to maintain independence or something else.

This book is for you if you answer "yes" to one or more of the following –

- I have competing demands on my time and don't have enough left to spend with my elderly relative.

- I feel confused and overwhelmed by the care system.

- I am worried about the increasing dependency of my elderly relative and don't know what to do.

- I live a long way from my elderly relative and am unable to visit as often as I would like or able to respond quickly in an emergency.

- I feel under pressure to make arrangements for my elderly relative who is being discharged from hospital.

- My elderly relative needs to go into a care home and I don't know which one to choose.

You will find this book helpful whether you are physically caring for your elderly relative, caring from a distance, co-ordinating and monitoring the care and support your relative is receiving from paid carers, or you just have the first inklings that your relative is going to need more help in the future.

Although writing from the perspective of a caring daughter supporting her parents, the information I provide will apply equally to any elderly relative, partner or friend. The book will provide an especially valuable resource for people who are not eligible for public funding and therefore do not have a social worker to help them navigate the complex care system.

HOW TO USE THIS BOOK

I recommend that you read the whole book to get maximum benefit from the information and advice. If you decide to dip into chapters as and when you need the information, be careful not to jump straight to finding solutions before having carefully identified the issues and challenges you need to resolve. If you are making life-changing decisions, these solutions will benefit from thorough consideration and research.

1. THE CARE SYSTEM AND ASSESSMENT MATTERS

In this chapter, I will continue to share my parents' journey and professional experiences. We will also look at the care system in England and the different type of assessments you might come up against, most of which determine eligibility criteria, which are rather like rules, to access social care or NHS funding and services.

The journey continues...

Following another fall, on this occasion breaking her wrist, Mum was temporarily admitted to a care home as she was unable to dress and undress or do the other things she had been able to do for herself before the fall. Whilst she was in the home her brother and sister both died on the same day. This upset her deeply, triggering depression and increased anxiety. It soon became clear that if Mum were to return home, she would need more care and support than Dad was able to give her. Following discussion with my brother and sister, I made a referral to Social Services.

The day after Mum returned home, a social worker arrived to carry out a care assessment and an assessment for the provision of community services. She also carried out a carer's assessment for my father. The result was that the Social Worker arranged for a care agency to visit Mum every morning to help her wash and dress and twice a week, to have a bath. In addition, she arranged for Mum to spend a week twice a year in a care home to give Dad a break from looking after her and also referred Mum to a welfare benefits adviser, to assess her ability to pay for services and ensure she was receiving all the benefits she was entitled to.

A referral was also made to the Falls Prevention Team for an assessment at our local hospital. This involved a physiotherapist, geriatrician and occupational therapist and resulted in a home visit to establish the equipment Mum needed to reduce her risk of falls, a list of exercises for her to do each day to strengthen her muscles and a referral to a community matron to assess her health needs.

I should point out that although all Social Services departments must assess anyone who has a disability, or appears to be in need of a community service, they all work differently and the terminology they use varies.

Reflecting on the time we got Social Services involved, it felt a bit like "death by assessment" with so many different professionals asking different and sometimes the same questions. As well as my mother having a problem with her memory, my father's short-term memory was also deteriorating, so being present at these various assessments was pretty important to ensure that my parents received the most appropriate help and equipment.

Healthcare in England

The Health & Social Care Act introduced a number of important changes in the NHS, which were introduced on 1st April 2013. Changes include:

- Disbanding Primary Care Trusts (PCTs) and strategic health authorities. In their place Clinical Commissioning Groups comprising of local GPs among others, will 'buy' healthcare for their local communities.

- A new body, NHS England will oversee the NHS.

- Responsibility for public health transferred to local authorities who will take the lead for improving the health of their local communities.
- Commissioning will take place through competitive tendering and NHS contracts will be opened to the private and voluntary sector.

However, none of these changes will affect how you access NHS services in England. The way you book your GP appointment, get a prescription, or are referred to a specialist, will not change. Healthcare will remain free at the point of use, funded from taxation and based on need and not the ability to pay.

Social Care in England

Care and support of older people in England has been a source of concern for successive governments. This is due to increasing unease about the implications of an ageing population, the affordability of long-term care and the lack of transparency and consistency in the current system.

This has resulted in the current Government changing the care system in the biggest overhaul since the introduction of the NHS in1948, with the intention of making it clearer and fairer.

The new Care Bill, published on the 10th of May 2013, brings together existing care and support legislation into a new, modern set of laws. The Care Bill will not be published until sometime in 2014 and then there will need to be regulations and guidance published to set out how it will be implemented. As always, the devil will be in the detail so we need to watch its introduction carefully.

Changes include:

- The reform to social care funding to be introduced from 2016 which puts a £72,000 cap on the 'reasonable' care costs incurred by people with eligible needs
- Raising the current means – tested threshold for people who are eligible for state funded social care from £23,520 to £118,000
- A new system of means-testing for community-based care services
- A national eligibility threshold for care and support
- New rights for carers which, for the first time, gives them the same rights to assessments and care services from local authorities as those they care for.

Needs Assessment for social care

Your relative may need services because of serious illness, physical disability, sensory impairment, mental health problems or loss of independence due to old age. Everyone has the right to request an assessment to discuss their needs, *including people who are not eligible for social care services and have to fund their own care.*

The Social Services assessment process consists of two interdependent elements. Firstly the level of need, and secondly, financial circumstances. Both benchmarks have to be met to be eligible for social care funding and support.

A Social Care Needs Assessment, sometimes called a Community Care Assessment, will usually take the form of a meeting to collect and record information to help understand more about your relative's circumstances and needs, along with how those needs impact on their ability to live a full and independent life. It is an opportunity for your relative to tell a social care professional about their circumstances and discuss their needs, with help if necessary.

A Needs Assessment will form part of the basis on which a decision will be made about your relative's eligibility to receive services from the local authority.

It also provides valuable information if your relative is to fund and arrange their own services at home, or in a care or nursing home.

The NHS and Social Services want to achieve one single process to cover health and social care assessment, but most are they way from achieving this aspiration.

One or more social care or health professionals may be involved, such as a social worker and occupational therapist, and they will spend time with your parent/relative, asking about their needs and circumstances. These may include issues of physical and mental health, personal care, safety, mobility and accommodation.

A Needs Assessment will help to determine:

- If a person is eligible for health and or social care funding and services
- What level of help and support the person needs
- What kinds of services are needed, from aids and adaptations in the person's home, to home care workers or residential care.

A social worker or care manager and sometimes an occupational therapist will assess your relative's level of need and what the level of risk is to their independence.

The eligibility thresholds are then applied to determine which categories of need they fall into.

Councils use a set of guidelines called 'Fair Access to Care Services Eligibility Criteria' to decide who should receive social care support in their area. These are set out by the Department of Health, and Social Services have to follow them.

There are four categories of need within the criteria: low, moderate, substantial and critical. Councils are able to decide which level of need they will meet for the eligibility threshold for their residents. Most councils have set this at *substantial* and only provide services for people assessed at the *substantial* and *critical* levels.

Due to the financial pressure councils are facing, many are restricting the number of people they are able to help and will only support those with a high level of need who require a significant amount of support.

The Assessment should show which needs are most important. It should also show the risks to your relative if they were not given any help. Your relative should be at the *centre* of the assessment process because they are the best person to understand their own needs and how to meet them.

Preparing for a needs assessment

You can play an important role in supporting your elderly relative to express their needs. Sometimes older people find it difficult to express how difficult certain tasks have become. If you are there with them you can provide moral support as well as offering gentle reminders about the problems they face.

Plan with your relative before the assessment and make notes. Ask them to think about what a bad day is like; what activities they have the most difficulty with; and what services and equipment might help. When answering questions during the Assessment, your relative should think about how they manage on a bad day without any help.

Alternatively, your parent can choose to have a friend or carer to help with their assessment or have an advocate to help them. Advocates can help people to secure their rights, represent their interests, find things out for them and help get the support they need.

What to do if you are unhappy with the Assessment

If you are unhappy with the assessment of your relative's needs for any reason, you can request a reassessment. If this is refused or you remain dissatisfied, you could consider making a complaint.

Financial assessment

The second element of the Assessment is the financial one. If your relative's level of need indicates that they may be eligible for social care funding, Social Services will carry out a means test. At the present time anyone with over £23,250 savings will not be eligible for funding and support from Social Services. However the level is due to increase in 2016 if the Care and Support Bill's intentions become law in 2014.

Financial assessment in practice

In my parents' situation, a finance officer from Social Services visited my parents at home to go through my mother's financial affairs with her and also make sure she was receiving all the welfare benefits she was entitled to. I was with them for the meeting, which was just as well as I had to find all their financial details, including bank statements, pension and benefit details, savings, investment and mortgage information, and Power of Attorney details. My parents had made arrangements for my brother, sister and me to act on their behalf if it became necessary.

Bob's Story

Bob's father had changed recently. His health had deteriorated, he was lethargic all the time and no longer wanted to meet his friends and play bowls at his club. Bob was so concerned he contacted his father's GP who advised him to refer the matter to Social Services. They asked Bob some questions and quickly identified that his father was not eligible for their services because his income put him above their financial threshold.

Bob asked me what he should do. I told him to request a Care Assessment for his father as he was entitled to one regardless of not being eligible for services. I suggested that he be present while it was carried out, to support his father and ensure he gave an accurate picture of his situation. This is important because older people typically over-estimate their abilities and play down the difficulties they are experiencing. I also asked Bob to be sure to ask for a copy of the Assessment, as it would provide information to help plan his father's care and support. Finally I suggested that he make an appointment for his father to see his GP for a thorough check up and medication review to see if there was a medical cause for his lethargy.

As Bob's father was not eligible for social care funding he would not have a social worker to help find the best and most appropriate care and support solutions for him. I find that it can be difficult for family members to do this on behalf of their relatives, as they often have little idea about the options available and how to access them. Without a good assessment, relatives can over-estimate the support their loved one needs. For example: seeing residential care as the best or only solution when their relative needs more care and support.

An occupational therapist (OT) will need to assess your relative for disability equipment and adaptations to their home. An OT assessment can take longer than other things to arrange as demands for their service are escalating, with the increasing demands of an ageing population.

Disability equipment and adaptations

An occupational therapist (OT) will need to assess your parent for disability equipment and adaptations to their home. An OT assessment can take longer than other things to arrange as demands for their service are escalating with the increasing demands of an ageing population.

Assessment for Continuing Healthcare (CHC)

NHS CHC is a package of services and support arranged and fully funded by the NHS for people with long-term health needs. This can be provided in the person's home in the community, or in a care home.

In a person's home, this means the NHS pays for healthcare, for example from a community nurse or specialist therapist, and for personal care including help with things like bathing and dressing. In a residential home, the NHS funds care or nursing home fees, including board and accommodation.

Eligibility for Continuing Healthcare support and funding is determined on the basis that someone's primary care need is a health need. A primary health need is determined by:

- The nature or type of condition or treatment
- The complexity – symptoms that are difficult to manage or control, or by their intensity – one or more needs which are so severe that they require frequent and skilled treatment
- The unpredictability – unexpected variable needs that are difficult to manage and present a risk to the individual or others.

If your relative doesn't qualify for Continuing Healthcare, Social Services will be responsible for assessing their care needs and providing services, if they are eligible.

Assessment for NHS-funded nursing care

Eligibility for NHS-funded nursing care, also called NHS Registered Nurse Care Contribution (RNCC) should not be considered for your relative until it has been agreed that they are not eligible for CHC and that a place in a nursing home is the best place for them.

Eligibility will be determined by assessment from a registered nurse. If eligible, NHS-funded nursing care will be paid as The Registered Nurse Care Contribution. This is a sum of money paid by the NHS to the nursing home for the care provided by a registered nurse. Your relative would still be responsible for paying the cost of their accommodation, board and personal care, although if their income and capital is limited they may be entitled to financial support from Social Services.

Other assessments

Other assessments your relative may come across are undertaken by home care and residential care providers. Home care providers need to determine if your parent's home is safe for their staff to work in and whether one or two staff are required. Residential managers are obliged to ensure their home can meet your parent's needs. In both cases, managers will visit your parent in their own home, in hospital or the residential care home they may be moving from.

Points to remember

- A person is entitled to an assessment of their needs even if they are not eligible for social care funding.
- Assessments can inform decision-making and help to determine the type and level of support your relative needs.
- Have a discussion with your relative beforehand to prepare for the assessment and make notes.
- If possible, be with your relative when they are being assessed to help them express their needs, provide support and ensure the information given accurately reflects their needs.
- Obtain and keep a copy of the assessment.

- The rules around financial assessment criteria will change after the Care Bill becomes law in 2014.

Did you know?

The primary carers of older people in Britain are most likely to be women in their 50s.

2. DIRECT PAYMENTS AND PERSONAL BUDGETS

In this chapter we will look at Direct Payments, Personal Budgets, which my parents used to obtain the services they chose to meet their assessed needs, and also at Personal Health Budgets. These payments are only available to people who have been assessed to meet the eligibility criteria for, social care from the local authority or NHS.

Direct Payments

For some years now Social Services have been under a duty to offer Direct Payments.

A Direct Payment works a bit like a benefits payment. It is a cash payment to an individual who uses it to pay people they have employed themselves to look after them, called Personal Assistants, or a care agency of his or her choice, to provide the support needed. A Direct Payment is one of the ways a personal budget can be paid.

Direct Payments are not a replacement of income and therefore do not affect any other benefits your parent may be receiving, and are not taxable.

Personal Budgets

A Personal Budget is an amount of money the local authority allocates to your relative's care based on its assessment of their needs.

A personal budget can give your relative more choice and control over how they live their life and enable care solutions to be more flexible and creative and tailored in a more personal way. They may, for example, want to attend a lunch club or go to the theatre instead of going to a day centre. They can still choose traditional support services, the important thing is that with a Personal Budget the choice is theirs, as long as it is used to support their social care needs.

The following story is a good illustration of how personalised and flexible Personal Budgets can be.

Susan's Story

Joe and Edna had been married for 60 years. They had brought up their three children and lived in the same house since the day they were married. They were active churchgoers and, as a retired teacher from a local school, Joe was well known in the area. It was important to them to both remain living in their own home and to remain part of their local community.

As Edna's health deteriorated, Joe's caring role began to take its toll on him and his own health needs required him to have care in his own right. Social Services provided a care package, which consisted primarily of 'pop in' calls throughout the day to check the couple were ok. Their family continued to support them to manage shopping and other domestic tasks.

Attending church and taking part in social activities became problematic and their diet deteriorated as it consisted of ready meals that neither of them really enjoyed. They regularly used the call button on their emergency alarm system day and night, which impacted on their family, and both were at high risk of falls.

After a few months their health deteriorated further. Joe had a fall and broke his hip while trying to help Edna in the bathroom. This meant he could no longer offer his wife any support. They both met Social Services criteria for residential care. However, they wished to remain living together in their own home.

With support from their daughter Susan, Joe and Edna decided to receive their Personal Budget as a Direct Payment. They purchased care from an agency that provided a 24-hour, live in carer and employed one of their other daughters as a personal assistant to cover the agency worker's time off.

Providing 24-hour care for Joe and Edna greatly improved their quality of life and reduced the risks associated with their health conditions, and vulnerability to exploitation. Joe no longer felt the burden of caring for Edna and, more importantly, Joe and Edna were able to remain living in their own home in a community they knew well. Edna was again able to participate in community activities and attended church regularly, something she had not been able to do for several years.

From the perspective of their family, having a Personal Budget enabled them to relax and feel that Joe and Edna were safe and well looked after. It also gave them the control and choice to help Joe and Edna find the best solution for them.

In addition to my parents being two of the first older people in the country to receive a Personal Budget, I was seconded to a Primary Care Trust (PCT) to lead the introduction of Personal Budgets for the NHS as part of the Department of Health's national Personal Health Budget Pilot Programme.

Personal Health Budgets

On 1st August 2013, the Direct Payment in Healthcare regulations came into force across England. This new legislation means that the NHS can offer personal health budgets as a direct payment, where the individual or their representative is given the money to organise the care themselves and, from April 2014, anyone receiving NHS continuing healthcare will have a right to ask for a Personal Health Budget.

Personal Health Budgets work in a similar way to the personal budgets that people are using for social care. At their heart is a personalised care plan, which sets out the health outcomes or goals to be met, the money available to meet them, and how that will be spent. As with social care, the amount of money in a Personal Health Budget will vary according to the person's assessed needs.

A Personal Health Budget can be used to meet a range of health needs, including physiotherapy, occupational therapy and equipment, complementary therapies, speech or language therapy, continence products, or wheelchairs and other mobility aids. Not all healthcare can be provided through a Personal Health Budget. For example, it will not be used to buy medication, pay for GP services and treatment, or for emergency/unplanned hospital care.

Points to remember

- People who are eligible for help from Social Services can request a Direct Payment or Personal Budget to choose and buy their own care and support.
- A Personal Budget using a Direct Payment enables people to have more choice and control over their social care.
- On 1st August 2013, the Direct Payment in Healthcare regulations came into force across England.
- From April 2014, anyone receiving NHS Continuing Healthcare will have a right to ask for a Personal Health Budget.

Did you know?

In March 2012, over half of the people receiving social care funding (432,000) chose to have a Personal Budget.

3. REVIEW AND COMPLAINT MATTERS

In this chapter we will look at what happens when your relative's needs are reviewed, how to complain if you are not satisfied and explore independent advocacy.

Reviews

If you or your elderly relative does not feel that all their needs were taken into account, or their needs change, you can ask for a reassessment from Social Services, even if your parent is funding their own care. If Social Services refuse a reassessment you can ask for a new assessment or make a complaint.

If your relative is supported by Social Services, their needs and the services provided by them will usually be reviewed after three months and annually thereafter. Unfortunately if your relative pays for their own care, the services they arrange and pay for will not be reviewed, neither will their needs be reviewed, unless they change and you request a reassessment. Some people engage an independent care consultant to carry out an annual review and ensure their relative's needs continue to be met and that they are getting the service they want, need and for which they are paying.

Making a complaint

Whether your relative receives care and support from the NHS, Social Services or an independent or private care provider, they have a right to be treated fairly and with respect. Sometimes things do not work out that way and you can feel dissatisfied either with the level, quality or type of service your relative receives or because they have been refused help or appropriate funding.

It is usually best to try and resolve the situation about which you are unhappy locally by speaking directly to the person involved in providing the care service or medical treatment. If this is not possible, or if the matter is serious, then it will need to be investigated as a complaint.

A single complaints system for all health and social care services now covers complaints against NHS hospitals, Clinical Commissioning Groups (CCGs), including GP practices, local authorities and independent providers. These services and organisations are required to set out their complaints procedure in a leaflet, so ask for a copy to begin with.

If you have concerns or wish to make a complaint about the quality of care your relative receives from the NHS, you can contact the Patient Advice and Liaison Service (PALS) at www.pals.nhs.uk to find your nearest office from their on-line directory.

If you are unhappy about Social Services, ring and ask to speak to their Complaints Officer who will advise you further.

Relatives can make a complaint themselves, or you can make it on their behalf. If the complaint relates to services provided by more than one organisation, they must co-operate with each other and ensure that you or your relative receives a co-ordinated response.

The organisation or service provider must investigate your complaint as quickly and efficiently as possible and keep you informed of progress. When the investigation has concluded they must send you a written response setting out how the complaint was considered and the conclusions they reached. They are also required to advise you of your right to take the complaint to the Local Government or Health

Service Ombudsman if you are not satisfied with the outcome.

If you have been refused NHS Continuing Healthcare you can ask for the decision to be reviewed. This process is separate from the NHS complaints procedure and you can ask the Continuing Healthcare Team in your area for information about their appeals process.

All professions have their own governing body and allegations of professional misconduct about a health or social care professional can be made to the body responsible for that individual. For example the General Medical Council for a doctor, General Social Care Council for a social worker and the Nursing and Midwifery Council for the nursing profession.

Here are some practical points to help you when making a complaint:

- Set up a file for the complaint.
- Follow the process outlined in the appropriate complaints leaflet.
- Put your complaint in writing.
- Make sure you put the word "complaint" in the subject heading.

- Keep focused on the complaint rather than how angry you are feeling.
- Keep a copy of all correspondence.
- Print a copy of emails and keep them together in the folder.
- Make a note of phone calls, along with the date and name of the person to whom you spoke.

If the concerns you have relate to any kind of abuse (for example neglect, theft or physical or emotional abuse) you should refer the matter to the Safeguarding Officer at Social Services *whether or not Social Services are funding your relative's care.* See also *Chapter 16,* Safeguarding Matters.

Ombudsmen

The Local Government Ombudsman provides a free service in England and deals with complaints about poor service, unfair treatment and administrative failures from Social Services. Ombudsmen have the powers of the High Court to gather information and then act to resolve justified complaints in a way that is fair to everyone involved.

Until fairly recently the only form of redress for people in privately funded care was through the care provider's own complaints procedure or by going to court. Now, if people who fund their own care, or members of their family, have suffered an injustice, the Ombudsman may be able to help. In most cases they will only consider a complaint once the care provider has had a fair opportunity to put things right.

If you wish to make a complaint to your Local Government Ombudsman you can contact the Advice Line on 0300 061 0614 or complete an on-line complaint form on their website www.llo.org.uk

If you disagree with the outcome of your complaint about NHS care after following their complaints procedure you can contact the Parliamentary and Health Service Ombudsman by telephoning 0345 015 4033 or via their website www.ombudsman.org.uk.

Carol's Story

A friend rang me one evening and she sounded angry. Her mother was in a care home, which she was funding herself and the home had just put up its fees substantially. To make matters worse there had been staffing problems and the quality of the meals had recently deteriorated. Carol said she didn't know what to do as it had taken months for her mother to settle at the home and she didn't want to move her again. I advised Carol to ask the home for a copy of their complaints procedure and follow it carefully. If the matters were not resolved I told her that she could now refer her concerns to the Local Government Ombudsman as the rules were changed in October 2010 to include self-funders.

I suggested she also check her mother's contract with the care home to establish whether the terms that were agreed are being breached. I said that if there was anything about the contract that she was not sure about she should take it to the Citizen's Advice Bureau (see chapter on resources for further details). Alternatively, she could try her local Trading Standards office. If the matter was still not resolved she may have to consider moving her mother, which hopefully would not be necessary.

If you remain dissatisfied

If your complaint is not resolved to you or your relative's satisfaction there are further steps you can take.

You can take the complaint to your relative's local MP or councillor. They hold surgeries in their constituency and can also be contacted by email or letter. You can also write to the government minister responsible for the public service you or your relative are concerned about.

It may be possible in some cases to challenge a decision made by a local authority Social Services or NHS department in a judicial review. The High Court hearing will look at whether the public body has followed the law correctly. A judicial review will only be agreed if all avenues of resolving the complaint have been tried and the issue was felt to be a misinterpretation of the law. You must be aware, however, that a judicial review can be very expensive if your relative does not qualify for legal aid.

It is also possible to take private legal action against a local authority. The process can be slow and expensive and should not be considered lightly. Do research the potential legal costs thoroughly before committing yourself or your relative and find a solicitor who has experience in community care law and services affecting older people. You will find some contacts to help you in *Helpful Resources*.

Independent Advocacy

In some situations you may find it helpful to have an independent advocate help your relative to resolve issues and clarify information between them and social and health care professionals. If your relative is unhappy about a situation or decision, an independent advocate will represent their rights and views and can discuss with them what outcome they would like. They can also attend meetings on your relative's behalf.

An independent advocate can speak on your relative's behalf to represent their views or support them to speak for themselves. They will not make decisions for your relative but will ensure that your relative has all the information they need to make an informed decision for themself. This can be helpful, to understand some of the complex information that organisations sometimes provide.

Having an independent advocate can be particularly helpful if you or your relative find it difficult to speak up for yourselves, if you find it difficult to stay calm and focused on the facts when emotions are running high, or if you feel unable to challenge the people involved.

Points to remember

- Only people who receive support from Social Services and the NHS will have their needs automatically reviewed.
- Your relative can make a complaint themselves or you can make it on their behalf.
- One system now covers complaints about the NHS, social care and independent providers and they are required to make information about their complaints procedure available to the public.
- People, who fund their own care and have an unresolved complaint, are now able to refer their concerns to the Local Government Ombudsman.
- If you suspect or are concerned about possible abuse, contact Social Services and ask to speak to the Safeguarding Coordinator. You can do this whether or not your relative receives support for their social care.

Did you know?

There were more than 100,000 complaints made against the NHS in 2009 – 2010.

4. HOSPITAL DISCHARGE MATTERS

In this chapter we will continue my parents' journey through the care system and explore the legal framework for hospital discharge, planned and unplanned admissions, the assessment, eligibility for NHS Continuing Healthcare funding, private hospital treatment, rehabilitation, convalescence, discharge to your parent's own home and discharge to a care or nursing home.

My father's memory has now deteriorated to be nearly as bad as my mother's. They have both experienced a significant hearing loss and have to wear two hearing aids. At least that's the plan, but more often than not Mum has lost one or both of hers. At the time of writing Dad has also lost his lower dentures, which had only been fitted two months ago. A great deal of time seems to be spent these days on looking for lost items. Some of the time with hilarious results!

I have set them up a health diary. This is so they can record their health concerns on a particular day and take the diary with them when they visit their GP. They use different colour pens to distinguish which parent is recording in the diary. I also plan the visits to the doctor with them before we go and jot down a few succinct points to sum up the reason for their visit. Their GP, in turn, records her advice and the prescribed treatment in the diary. The doctor said she wished all families planned appointments that way as it enables her to diagnose her patient more quickly and accurately.

The legal framework for hospital discharge

Your relative cannot be discharged from hospital until they are medically fit and are formally discharged by a named doctor or consultant. Well that's the theory, but the practice can sometimes feel very different!

Every hospital should have its own discharge policy based on government guidance. This policy will set out how the hospital will ensure that your relative's discharge is arranged safely. You can obtain a copy from the ward manager or the Patient Advice and Liaison Service (PALS) at their local hospital.

If your relative already receives care and support or are likely to need it when they return home, discharge planning is likely to begin at the pre-admission assessment and be reviewed throughout their stay in hospital. The process that must be followed before people can be discharged from a hospital stay for planned treatment, or surgery, or because they were admitted in an emergency, is set out in The Community Care (Delayed Discharges etc.) Act 2003.

This Act requires hospitals to advise Social Services if they believe that someone is likely to need care and support when they leave hospital, either in their own home or in a care or nursing home. The hospital must contact Social Services again as soon as the discharge date has been confirmed. The Act does not apply to palliative care, mental health care, non-acute care in a community hospital or people in an English hospital who live in Northern Ireland, Scotland or Wales.

Hospital staff should speak to your relative in advance about the date they are planning to discharge them. They must also make sure that your relative has transport home as well as any medication they will need when they get home.

Practice between hospitals is likely to vary on the procedure they follow if care and support has not been arranged by the anticipated discharge date. Sometimes the hospital will move the person to a temporary care home while home care support is being arranged or a vacancy arises in a home they have chosen. This is known as transitional care and the hospital must advise the family if it intends to make transitional arrangements.

Finding out how to navigate the care system is more difficult when we are responding to the immediate demands of a crisis and having to make decisions in a hurry. At this time, major life changing decisions are often made on the basis of little information, and relatives mostly have little idea about where to seek information and advice.

It costs less to keep someone in a care home than keeping them in hospital and people can feel anxious and put under pressure to move their loved one into a care home when their relative would rather return home, or move into a home they have chosen themselves. People who fund their own care are further disadvantaged by not having a social worker to help them navigate the complex care system and

Social Services rely heavily on relatives to do this for them. If a person who funds their own care is unable to return home without support and does not have a relative to help them, Social Services will usually place them in a care home.

Sarah's Story

Sarah became worried when her mother fell and broke her hip. Since her father passed away a few months before, her mother had become more dependent on her and Sarah was struggling to cope with a demanding job and looking after her disabled husband. Putting her mother into a care home seemed the obvious solution but Sarah knew that her mother had a fear of being put into a home and had always said that she only wanted to leave the home she had lived in all her married life, in a box.

As the time of her mother's discharge grew nearer, Sarah felt the discharge team at the hospital were steering her mother towards residential care with haste and before other options had been explored. In addition to the house she lived in, her mother had some modest savings and had been told that she was not eligible for social care funding.

Sarah had been given a list of care homes and in a nutshell, left to get on with it.

Sarah felt angry that just because her parents had been careful with their money after they retired her mother was denied a social worker to help with making a life changing decision. Sarah felt that just being given a list of care homes was not helpful and asked me to help her find the right home for her mother.

We carefully went through the assessment of her mother's needs that the discharge team had given Sarah and I made suggestions for putting together a care package so that her mother could return home. We made a plan of what we wanted to achieve and I told Sarah that the NHS has a responsibility to provide a rehabilitation service free of charge for up to four weeks after discharge, with the aim of helping her mother to regain her independence.

Sarah's mother was discharged two days later with a rehabilitation package in place. While it was being implemented, Sarah and I worked together to make arrangements to implement the longer-term care plan we had made.

A good discharge should be a process rather than an isolated event, undertaken by a multi-disciplinary team. Members of the team may include social workers, nurses, physiotherapists, occupational therapists and speech therapists.

Planned admissions

If your relative has to go into hospital for an operation or other medical treatment, it will help if you are able to go with them for their pre-admission assessment. As well as providing support, you will also be able to find out about the proposed tests or surgery, the anticipated length of stay, what can be expected during their stay and what the likely impact of the surgery or treatment will be on your relative's independence and future needs. If your relative is not given this information it is important that you ask for it. You should also discuss your relative's expectations early on so that misunderstandings can be avoided. Also ask how you and your relative can be involved in decisions about their hospital care.

Unplanned admissions

If your relative's stay in hospital was not planned it is important that you start working with staff to plan their discharge as soon as their condition has been diagnosed and a treatment plan is in place.

As both my parents have a problem with their memory and get in a muddle when they are feeling anxious, I have written down their details for emergencies – such as an emergency admission to hospital or to give paramedics when they arrive to get Mum off the floor following a fall. Paramedics have to fill in a form each time they are called and appreciate the time saved by having the information they need close at hand. Here are the headings I use that you may find helpful for your own elderly relative.

Information in case of emergency

Full name_____

Likes to be called _____

Address _____

_____

_____

Date of birth _____

Name and contact details for next of kin

_____

_____

Telephone _____

Name and address of GP _____

_____

_____

Condition/disability _____

Prescribed medication _____

Best way to communicate _____

Issues to be aware of _____

Discharge assessments

Your relative has a right to an assessment on leaving hospital, whether or not they are funding their own care and support. See *Chapter 1* for more information about assessment.

A range of professionals may be involved in the assessment depending on the complexity of your relative's needs. These may include, an occupational therapist to advise on any aids and adaptations or equipment your parent may need when they return home, physiotherapist, dietician, speech therapist, specialist nurse (such as for diabetes or mental health). A Social Worker should also be involved if your parent is likely to need, or continue to need, support from Social Services. It is important to let staff know if your relative has sight or hearing problems so they can ensure that your relative is fully involved in discussions and that any associated needs are recognised during their assessment.

You should know who is co-ordinating your parent's assessment and for ensuring agreed timescales are met. If you are unhappy with the assessment you should talk to this person about it and consider making a complaint if they are unable to resolve the matter.

NHS Continuing Healthcare funding

The issue of paying for care is a minefield and can be very stressful for people. If you believe that your relative should not be funding his or her own care do not agree to a discharge from hospital. If they appear likely to be eligible for NHS Continuing Healthcare funding, NHS staff have to take reasonable steps to ensure that an assessment for this funding is carried out before they advise Social Services of their potential need for community care services. See *Chapter 1* for further information.

If your relative has a primary health need, for example a major stroke, and the hospital say they are unable to do anymore for them, make sure you do not agree to a discharge for your relative until you have been given written confirmation, that the NHS will fund the nursing home placement.

Private hospital treatment

People can choose which hospital they wish to be treated in and your relative may want to choose a hospital nearer to you. They may also choose an independent or private hospital if they can meet the cost or have private health insurance.

Importantly, if your relative chooses an independent or private hospital, it is essential that you both think seriously about the services that are available before and after your relative's discharge because the Delayed Discharge Act does not always cover private hospitals. This means they do not have a duty to inform Social Services that your relative may need support when they leave hospital. This includes arranging healthcare services.

In this situation, you or your relative needs to ask the person in charge of their care, when they are first admitted to hospital, to contact Social Services on their behalf before they leave.

If the NHS has arranged your relative's stay in an independent hospital, the NHS will retain overall responsibility. The hospital must, therefore, comply with the Act by notifying Social Services that your relative is in need of support and identify any health service help they require.

Rehabilitation

When your relative is ready to leave hospital they may be offered a period of rehabilitation. This is a health service provided to enable people regain the maximum level of independence and enable them to resume living at home.

Rehabilitation is usually provided following a heart attack, stroke, hip fracture, pneumonia or an acute attack of a chronic health problem and treatment can be provided by a longer stay in hospital or rehabilitation unit. Services can include occupational therapy, physiotherapy and speech therapy.

Rehabilitation services vary across the country, so find out about your relative's local eligibility criteria by talking to the medical consultant or nursing staff.

Intermediate Care

Intermediate care, sometimes called reablement, is a range of services designed to help people remain independent, regain their independence, or enable them to return home from hospital. It can be provided by Social Services or the NHS and might be provided in a person's own home, a care home or day hospital.

Intermediate care can be provided for up to six weeks but frequently for less. It is provided free of charge by the NHS and sometimes by Social Services. If your relative is assessed as needing an item of equipment under £1,000 to return home safely, it must be provided free of charge.

If your relative does not meet their health authority's criteria for Continuing Healthcare, rehabilitation or intermediate care, Social Services will be responsible for assessing their needs – whether or not they are eligible for Social Services funding. However, if your relative is not eligible for funding, relatives are expected to arrange any services they need to return home.

Convalescence

Obviously an acute hospital is not the ideal environment for your relative to recover from an operation or illness but the harsh reality of returning home can be a very difficult time, especially for someone elderly.

Convalescent homes are few and far between and your relative may struggle to find a short-term vacancy in a care home at the time when support is most needed. However, I found that there are a number of convalescent and care homes associated with particular professions or charities that offer a great service to their members, although your relative may have to travel a fair distance.

After my father was discharged from a six week hospital stay ten years ago, I found and arranged for both my parents to go into a convalescent home for a couple of weeks. The home was wonderful. They grew their own vegetables and the food was fantastic because a nutritious balanced diet is an important part of a person's recovery. It was also important for my father to have a period of being looked after himself before resuming his caring role for my mother. The staff were wonderful.

The financial effect of a hospital admission

Some of your relative's benefits may be withdrawn after they have been in hospital for a certain number of weeks so it's worth checking them out. They include:

1. Attendance Allowance.
2. Constant Attendance Allowance.
3. Pension Credit.
4. Housing Benefit.
5. Council Tax Benefit.

Points to remember

- Your elderly relative should not be discharged from hospital until they are considered medically fit for discharge.

- Discharge planning should begin as soon as possible and Social Services should be made aware if your relative will need care and support when they return home.

- Your relative is entitled to an assessment when being discharged from hospital, whether or not they are funding their own care.

- If your relative is going into a private or independent hospital, you both need to consider the services available before and after their discharge.

Did you know?

Two thirds of NHS patients are aged sixty-five and over but they receive only two-fifths of total expenditure.

5. CARE PLANNING MATTERS

In this chapter we will rejoin the journey with my parents, explore the importance of care planning and how to find out about services. Although my parents receive funding from the state, the principles of their situation can equally be applied to people who are funding their own care. They are also Personal Budget holders – they just miss out the middle-man!

In 2006 my parents were among the first older people in the country to be given a Personal Budget managed through a Direct Payment from Social Services. Both my parents' health was deteriorating and although Dad's needs were not as substantial as Mum's, he was given a small budget of his own to take account of his significant caring role.

The care plan produced by a social worker required a home-care agency to provide personal care for my mother every morning to help her get washed and dressed. The care worker would arrive any time between 9.00am and midday, which was much to my father's irritation as the irregular times interrupted their daily routine. The care workers were only permitted to undertake personal care tasks and nothing more.

When Dad needed a break to recharge his batteries, the only option was for Mum to go into a care home. It was a home that the council had a contract with and the room was barely big enough to swing a cat and had no TV. Other than the times my mother was hospitalised, my parents hadn't spent a night apart since they were married and my mother hated it.

Having a Personal Budget made a huge difference to them both.

Care planning with my parents

First we made our own Care Plan showing Social Services how we wanted to spend the money my parents had been allocated. This involved me asking careful questions and watching and listening to their response. We then established the outcomes or goals they wanted to achieve.

Here is what we came up with

- Consistent care workers who arrived at the same time each day.

- Flexible care arrangements, which included daily living tasks as well as personal care and allowed time for reassuring my mother when she became depressed, anxious or had a nightmare during the night.

- Having someone not only take my mother to medical appointments, but also go in with her to remind her what she was there for and report back what was said.

- Respite care in different settings, with Dad going with Mum for some of the breaks.

- Finding a solution to reduce the accidents Mum had as a result of forgetting to turn her catheter tap off when she emptied it.

- Ensuring that Mum took the correct medication at the right time.

We discussed broad options before I researched ways to achieve the goals my parents had identified. It is important to note that the package cost no more than that arranged by the social worker for Mum before my parents had a Personal Budget.

Here is what my parents proposed, which was approved by Social Services:

- Employ two personal assistants (PAs). Employing staff directly is cheaper than paying an agency so we could have more hours for our money. I also agreed to provide care myself at weekends when higher rates would otherwise have to be paid. This enabled my father to have his own PA for a few hours a week and my mother to have more hours of support to include housework, shopping, ironing and escorting her to medical appointments, in addition to personal care.

- My mother would attend a small, local day centre to provide her with mental stimulation and a regular weekly break for my father from caring for her.

- While Mum was at the day centre (which we called "a club" as she didn't want to go to a day centre) a PA would take Dad for a walk. This not only provided him with physical exercise, he could have a coffee or a pint while they were out and enjoy "boy's talk" as a change from talking to and reassuring my anxious mother.

- A variety of arrangements would provide respite breaks for both my parents, including a stay at a small hotel near friends in Bournemouth, with a local care agency providing personal care for my mother, and a luxury care home run and subsidised by the RAF that provides respite breaks(my father was in the RAF police during the war). Once a year my mother would also go into a care home on her own to give my father a complete break and to provide a familiar setting, should my father become ill or pass away before her.

- Medication dispensed weekly by the pharmacist into a monitored dose container that vibrated and rang an alarm each time my mother's medication was due.

- A small piece of technical equipment fixed to the wall in the bathroom where Mum emptied her catheter. This included a motion sensor and as she turned to empty her catheter the movement triggered a pre -recorded message which reminded her to turn the tap off. Dad and I alternated to change the tone or wording of the message slightly each week and avoid Mum becoming used to the message and ignoring it.

Care plans

The care plan (sometimes called a support plan) is a document, which states what a person's needs are and how it is proposed to meet those needs.

If it has been decided that, following an assessment, your relative is eligible to receive support services provided by Social Services in their own home or in a care home funded by Social Services, they should receive a written care plan that clearly states their individual needs and goals and how they will be met. The care plan will specify the following:

- Your relative's eligible needs.
- What care or equipment is needed.
- Who is responsible for making sure the care plan is carried out.
- What people have agreed to do.
- When they will do it.
- Who is responsible for making sure everything is going according to plan.

Your relative has the right to receive a copy of the plan. If they don't, you should ask for one. If you are unhappy with the plan and feel that it does not accurately reflect your relative's needs this should be raised with the person who wrote it.

If your relative has complex needs and has been assessed as ineligible for Social Services, or has chosen not to ask them for help, it is important that you make a care plan with them or ask a professional to help you. This is not, of course, necessary if all your relative needs is a single, straightforward service, like shopping or gardening.

Meg's Story

Meg's eighty-five year old mother Violet had severe arthritis, a heart condition and was showing early signs of dementia. She had a care package, which was funded by Social Services, and Meg and her sister supported Violet on Sundays. When Social Services changed their criteria, Violet's funding was reduced due to the financial pressures on Social Services. Following reassessment by her social worker, shopping and a monthly visit to her sister were no longer funded. Also, Meg's request for support for her mother during the night in case she wandered into the road, was refused, being considered a low risk because Violet had never actually left her home at night. Here is how we arranged to meet Violet's un-met needs.

Meg would take her laptop and mobile broadband when she visited Violet each week. Then she could go through what shopping her mother needed with her and place an order on-line.

Meg had a demanding job, so was unable to take Violet to see her sister during the week when it was more convenient for her aunt. Meg arranged to support her mother on one Saturday afternoon each month, which freed up some of the care worker's time so that she could then take Violet to see her sister during the week.

Meg bought a *Wander Minder* and placed it by Violet's front door. This is a small unit with a motion sensor and timer that can be set to emit a pre-recorded message at night telling her mother that it is unsafe for her to go out (the same kind of device I used for mum's catheter challenge). Meg also purchased a *contact mat*, which has a battery-operated transmitter designed to be placed under the front door mat. When stepped on, the mat triggers the transmitter and alerts the carer. As she lived nearby, Meg could respond quickly if her mother tried to leave the house.

Time and time again I hear about people who fund their own services being given a list of care homes or home care agencies and being left to get on with it. All too often this has life-changing consequences, such as giving up their home and going into a care home without exploring other available options. If you or your relative is aware of their entitlement to a needs assessment, regardless of whether they fund their own services, or they have been in hospital and been given an assessment of their needs, this can be used to inform the care plan.

Here are some questions to help you develop a care plan with your relative:

1. What is the most important thing in the world to you? This is the overall goal such as: "To remain living in my own home".

2. What results will we see when the needs identified in the assessment have been met?

3. What needs to happen to enable you to achieve this? (Smaller goals such as: "To maintain personal hygiene/to take the correct medication regularly/maintain a healthy diet/maintain the use of my left arm" etc.)

4.   What do you need to do to achieve these goals? For example, have help with my personal care, taking medication, shopping, food preparation and doing the exercises I was shown.

5.   What support do you need for these? (Try and help them to think "outside the box" such as someone could help them to shop on-line which would maintain their independence and could cost less)

6.   What will it cost?

7.   How will you ensure that you are kept safe?

8.   Who will be responsible for arranging the support to implement the plan?

9.   When will the plan be implemented?

10.   What contingencies can be put in place for emergencies?

Points to remember

A care plan identifies what your relative wants to achieve and sets out a plan to achieve it.

- Your relative should be given a copy of their care plan if they are receiving support from Social Services.

- If your relative is not eligible for support from Social Services and they have complex care and support needs, you should make a plan with them or ask a professional to help you.
- An assessment of your relative's needs can be used to inform their care plan.

Did you know?

Small things can make a big difference to an older person.

6. ACCOMMODATION MATTERS

In this chapter we will continue my parents' journey and consider the various living options that are available to older people.

Both my parents are becoming more dependent and as their ability to function decreases, my involvement has increased. It is difficult to see two people you care about, who have always been very independent, becoming more dependent and frustrated by having to rely more and more on others. I have found it difficult to watch Dad struggle with the mysteries of the remote control for the TV and to understand the most basic tasks, when he had always been the one to translate complex instructions for the latest piece of electrical equipment for me.

Telephone calls to deal with emergencies, typically about Mum having a fall, were increasing and I was still working full-time. After a particularly difficult week I knew something had to be done. The solution I came up with was to arrange a personal response service. This was provided by Mum and Dad's community alarm provider and was an "add-on" service to their existing system. From now on, if Mum had a fall or either of them had any kind of emergency, they could summon help by pressing their alarm and my work would not be interrupted.

The service was excellent. The call centre was given information about them both. The staff responded calmly to calls, by asking which of them had the problem and what it was. They would then send the most appropriate help, for example if Mum had a fall they would send an ambulance. For non-medical emergencies they would send a roving support worker. If they considered the matter to be serious, they would also contact me.

If your relative is no longer able to manage in their own home but is not ready or willing to move into a care home there are a number of alternatives.

Social Services and the Primary Care Trust have a duty to produce information about the services they provide for your relative's area. This will range from information leaflets up to and including strategic plans, which are called Community Care Plans or Long-Term Care Charters. These show how Social and NHS services will meet the needs of their local population.

The help and support our relatives may require, as they grow older, can range from the installation of a stair lift in their own home, to permanent residence in a high dependency nursing home. There is, of course, a whole range of requirements in between.

Caring for your elderly relative may involve them physically living with you and you acting as their primary carer, or supporting them in their own home. Both can be demanding. If your relative maintains their independence and stays in their own home, the level of support they need may be quite high. It may be that your relative needs professional care, in which case your role as a carer is one step removed and you become the co-ordinator of the care provision. Your relative's care needs may vary over relatively short periods, for example after a stay in hospital, or their need may only be temporary whilst their usual carer is on holiday. Whatever their individual needs, there is a huge range of care services, support organisations and voluntary groups to help them. Very often the problem is that we are not aware of just what is available and how our relative might access it.

Here are some of the accommodation and care options available to your elderly relative and how to access them.

Having a relative move in to live with you

In my experience, an elderly parent or other relative moving in to live with their adult children is usually a response to some kind of crisis in their life. Other reasons include feelings of guilt about putting their parent in a care home or the view that it will be more convenient than looking after them from a distance.

I cannot stress enough how important it is to think carefully beforehand about the decision to move your relative in with you. While the arrangement can work well for some, I have known many people who regretted their decision and, once it has been made, it can be very difficult to change the arrangement. While Social Services will provide some support, if your parent meets their criteria, such as help with personal care and occasional respite to give you a break, with limited resources they will be reluctant to fund a care home placement as an alternative.

Your relative's needs are likely to increase as they become older and they may become incontinent and or confused. If they have been independent all their life, they are going to find the transition difficult and feel a burden on you whatever you try and do to avoid it.

I would advise you and your parent to get separate legal advice and consider having a formal agreement drawn up. This may sound over the top but you will be pleased you did if things do not go according to plan in the future.

Here are some questions to ask yourself before making your decision:

- How would your relative moving in impact on you and your family?
- Have you got sufficient space for them to have their own living area and bathroom? If not how will you and they entertain visitors and avoid needing the bathroom at the same time?
- Will you need to have your home adapted?
- How will you arrange meal times? Will your parent eat with you and your partner? What about when your children visit or you want to entertain friends?
- How will finances be worked out?
- How will you feel about the possibility of having strangers (carers) increasingly coming into your home?

- What would need to happen for the arrangement to work out well?
- What would need to happen for the arrangement to become unacceptable?

Jane's story

Since her husband died, Jane's mother had become increasingly dependent. She lived in a flat about ten minutes' drive away and Jane was finding it difficult to find the time to visit her on top of a demanding job. Jane is a widow and as her sister only visited their mother occasionally, she knew she could not rely on her when considering long-term care options for their mother.

Jane lived in a bungalow and her mother was financially independent. After careful consideration Jane suggested that her mother fund an extension to her own bungalow and move in with her, on condition that she would cook her mother's meals but would not provide personal care. Her mother agreed, the extension was built and she moved in with Jane.

After the first year, things began to get on top of Jane. Her mother became less concerned with personal hygiene and clearly needed help with her personal care but refused help from "an outsider". As soon as Jane came home from work her mother bombarded her with questions, ignoring Jane's pleas to switch off from work first. Social Services were unable to help with respite care to give Jane a break because her mother was over their financial threshold and the situation was almost at breaking point when Jane asked me for help.

Jane told me that what she needed most in order to continue caring for her mother was regular breaks. We explored options and agreed that her mother could have regular breaks in the Royal Air Force home my parents used, as her father had also been in the RAF and her mother would meet the cost herself. Her mother would also attend a retirement club run twice a week by a local voluntary organisation, who would also provide transport.

This improved things for a couple of years. However her mother's health deteriorated and she continued to refuse help with her personal care. The situation had reached breaking point when Jane's mother was taken ill and admitted to hospital where she unfortunately died a week later.

Homeshare

A useful and lesser-known option to consider is that in some parts of the country there are schemes called *Homeshare* that arrange for a younger person to move in with an elderly person to look after them in return for their board and lodgings. You can find out if there is a *Homeshare* scheme in your relative's area by checking out the website for *Homeshare International*, details of which are in the *Resources* section.

Moving to a more suitable property

It might be worth your elderly relative moving to a new home without stairs, in a more convenient location, in better repair, easier to maintain or without a garden. A range of housing options are available, designed to meet the needs of older people with disabilities and mobility problems. Generally the housing is designed and built to make everything accessible to wheelchair users.

Moving to a home where help, support or care is at hand

There is a wide range of housing built specially for the needs of older people, from traditional sheltered accommodation to retirement villages. More and more "schemes" have care staff discreetly at hand to provide assistance when needed for more frail or vulnerable old people. These include:

Sheltered Housing

There are a number of different types of sheltered housing schemes but basically accommodation and care and support are provided separately. They offer contained accommodation with communal space and a manager or warden, as well as providing 24-hour emergency assistance through a call alarm system. Sheltered housing enables people to live independently without being isolated, with the confidence of having access to help in an emergency.

Sheltered Social Housing

Local councils and housing associations provide rented sheltered housing, which are non-profit making organisations that provide housing for people on low incomes. If your parent owns their own property they are unlikely to be able to rent a flat in one of these sheltered housing schemes unless there are extenuating circumstances. If rented accommodation is being considered, it is worth checking with the Housing Department at their local council.

Private rented sheltered housing

Private sheltered housing is quite rare but the Elderly Accommodation Council (see *Helpful Resources*) may be able to help you.

Private ownership schemes

Private schemes seem to be springing up everywhere to meet the growing demands of our elderly population. However, they can be expensive and on-going service charges high. It is also important that your parent only considers buying from a builder who is registered with the National House Building Council (NHBC) and is covered by its sheltered housing code. Once schemes have been built, they are usually managed by a separate management company that provides a scheme manager and property maintenance. It is important that you research the company well and be sure to get independent professional advice on your parent's rights and responsibilities. The managing agent can make the difference between a good and bad living experience for your parent so time spent on checking them out will be a good use of your time.

Questions to ask when buying a property in a sheltered housing scheme:

- Is the scheme manager a member of a recognised trade organisation such as the Association of Retirement Housing Managers (ARHM)?
- What are the service charges, utility bills, ground rent and council tax costs?
- Are there plans to increase the service charge?
- What is the company's record of increasing service charges?
- Can the older person remain in their flat if their health deteriorates?
- Under what circumstances would someone be asked to leave?
- Is there enough storage space?
- What are the arrangements for emergencies?

- What are the communal facilities like?
- Is accommodation for guests available?
- Are pets allowed?
- Are social activities organised?

Extra Care Schemes

Extra care schemes are increasingly offering an alternative to residential care and aimed at less mobile people and wheelchair users.

Schemes usually consist of flats with an accessible lounge/diner, bedroom, bathroom and kitchenette. They have 24-hour care, support staff and a warden or manager on site. Some schemes include the provision of one meal a day in an on-site restaurant and cleaning services.

Different schemes offer various packages of personal and domestic care services that may include domestic assistance, practical help and support, personal care, and nursing care and assistance in an emergency. Basic staff cover is typically provided by the scheme, although your relative may be able to purchase additional personal care and practical help from an agency or use someone they have employed themselves. Housing or voluntary associations in partnership with Social Services usually develop extra care schemes, although an increasing number of private developers are coming on the scene.

Close Care

Some residential care providers also provide independent flats or bungalows on the same site as the care home. These schemes are called Close Care sheltered housing. An Extra Care or Close Care option will offer your parent more privacy and independence than a care home.

You can find out whether an Extra Care or Close Care scheme is available in your parent's area by contacting their local housing department.

Retirement villages

Retirement villages are a relatively new concept adopted from the United States of America. They are typically larger developments of 100 units or more and are growing in popularity in the United Kingdom. As they are a fairly new concept, the design and layout of the properties are more user-friendly than older housing options.

Retirement villages offer independent bungalows and apartments together with a range of social and leisure facilities and shops together with flexible levels of care and support that can be adapted to the needs of residents. Schemes may offer properties to buy, to rent or on a shared ownership basis. The range of facilities and services will vary significantly across different providers but most offer residential and nursing home care on the same site.

Retirement villages enhance the range of housing options available to older people, with a combination of independence and security together with opportunities for an active social life, all on one site. They also provide the opportunity to move from supported living to residential or nursing home care while maintaining the same friendship group within the same geographical location.

Whatever option suits your relative, make sure you share the decision making with them. They don't want to sit on the sidelines in their own life and be treated as a child. Ask them whether they would like to stay in their own home; if not, where they would like to live and how they would like their care handled. Encourage them to be open and candid with you about their choices and then listen carefully to their desires and concerns.

Gifted Housing Service

One of the lesser known solutions for accommodation is the Gifted Housing Service. If your relative owns their home and is worried about the costs and responsibility of maintaining it, they might wish to consider donating their property to the Gifted Housing Service run by *Age UK*. In return for donating their property, *Age UK* would help them to maintain their independence at home by supporting them in a number of ways including organising and paying for repairs, paying council tax and water rates and should they need it, contributing towards the cost of care either in their own home or in residential care. You can find their contact details in the *Resources* section.

Points to remember

There is a large range of living options to meet your relative's needs including:

- Moving to a more suitable home
- Having a relative move in with you
- Homeshare
- Sheltered housing
- Extra care schemes

- Close care
- Retirement villages
- Gifted Housing Service

Make sure you involve your relative in making the decision about where they want to live.

Did you know?

Nearly one in five people in the United Kingdom will live to see their 100th birthday.

7. ENVIRONMENT AND EQUIPMENT MATTERS

In this chapter we will look at the things we can do to help our elderly relatives remain in their own home for as long as possible; the part equipment played in helping my parents live safely in their own home; and a home safety checklist we used in the Homecare service, for which I was responsible.

Most older people want to stay in their home for as long as possible, but as they become older it can become harder to manage. This can be due to a disability or health problems, but with simple adaptations and equipment, your relative may be able to stay in their home for longer. Some examples are alterations to the building such as widening a door for a wheelchair, the installation of a stair lift, or a ramp to the front or back door. They could also include larger work, such as level-access showers, having an extension built or the kitchen adapted.

You can ask Social Services to arrange an assessment by an occupational therapist to clarify how your relative's needs can best be met. Once their eligibility is confirmed by an assessment, equipment is provided free of charge up to £1,000 if your relative is on a low income without a large amount of savings, assistance with more expensive adaptations, such as providing access to rooms, widening doors and installing ramps or providing an air conditioning or heating system, may be provided through a Disabled Facilities Grant (DFG) administered by your relative's local council. However, you need to be aware that DFGs can take several months to be processed.

If your relative is not eligible for a DFG, there are a number of charitable and benevolent societies that offer grants to people from certain professions, the armed forces or who simply need timely assistance, like my father with his urgent need for a walk-in shower. A good place to go for a directory of such organisations is *Turn2us*, for which details are given in *Helpful Resources*.

As our relatives become older, their senses of smell, sight, hearing and touch change and their ability to perform even basic tasks can present a challenge. It is therefore very important to ensure that their home environment is safe. Let's take a walk around a house and I will point out the things we need to consider, that I learned about when I managed a homecare service. At the end of this chapter you will also find a home safety checklist to help you do a safety audit of your elderly relative's home.

Access

If your elderly relative is finding it difficult to get in and out of their property, there are things that can be done to make it easier. This applies to their main access, usually the front door, their back door and access to the garden if they have one.

If they are finding it difficult climbing a step or steps up to the front door they could have a rail installed and set in concrete. Alternatively they could have a smaller grab rail at the door to help them step over the threshold safely.

If your relative uses a wheelchair they may need to have a ramp installed. Ramps have to meet a number of design standards to ensure they are safe in all conditions. You can also get a portable ramp if your relative has someone who can install and remove it afterwards. In some circumstances, for example if there isn't much space around the house, a wheelchair lift can provide access.

Answering the door

If your relative is finding it difficult to get to the front door when someone calls, there are a number of options. The most important things to consider are safety and security and you should thoroughly investigate options before making changes.

Your relative can have a door-entry intercom installed. This can either be one where they can talk to their visitor via an intercom link and then walk to the front door, or one where there is a push-button they can press to let the person in. Alternatively they can have a key safe installed, where the key is held in a secure box by their front door. Only people who have been given the code can open the door. My parents had a key safe installed and it has proved very useful for their carers to gain entry without Mum and Dad having to open the door for them.

Getting up and down stairs

If your relative is finding it difficult to get up and down stairs they may be able to have an extra banister rail or they can have a stair-lift installed to make it easier for them. A stair-lift is a mechanical seat that moves up and down along a rail attached to the stairs. There are many different types of stair-lift and they are not cheap. It would therefore be advisable to seek advice from an occupational therapist (OT) before purchasing one. You can contact your relative's Social Services department to access an OT.

The kitchen

Make sure your relative can reach everything in cupboards to avoid excessive reaching or climbing on a chair. Preparing food can mean your relative has to stand for long periods while preparing food. If they have difficulty standing you could get them a perching stool which enables them to have a near standing position while supporting them at the same time.

You need to check that appliances are in good working order and if they haven't got one already, get them a small basic microwave (for heating frozen meals) and place it where the keypad can be read easily.

The bathroom

Grab rails can be installed by the bath and toilet. Your relative may also need one on the wall outside the bath to help them get in and out. They may benefit from a raised toilet seat or a frame with arms around the toilet. Their bathroom cabinet may need to be repositioned to avoid unnecessary stretching.

Make sure your relative has a non-slip mat in their bath, or shower strips in the shower to prevent slips and falls. It may be necessary to have the bath removed so they can have a walk in shower or wet room.

The bedroom

If your relative is finding it difficult to manage stairs you may want to consider a stair-lift, or if they have a cloakroom, moving their bedroom downstairs. If neither of these is possible they may need to consider moving to accommodation that has level access.

A lamp should be placed near the bed so that your relative can have some light when using the bathroom during the night. You can now get lamps with a motion sensor, so the light comes on automatically when they get up in the dark. They need not be expensive. I managed to get my mother a light with a motion sensor to go over the bed for under £10.

Hallways and stairs

Your relative's hall and stairway should have handrails and lights with easy to access switches. Their stair carpet should be free of wrinkles and worn areas, which could cause them to trip and fall.

Other areas

- Garages should have a door that is easy to open.
- Windows should be easy to open but have a secure locking system on the ground floor.
- Smoke alarms should be fitted on each floor and the battery replaced once a year.
- A carbon monoxide detector should be placed near gas appliances.

Moving around your relative's home

If your elderly relative is having difficulty moving around their home it is important that you consider the risks related to particular floor surfaces, clutter and lighting.

If they need their essential facilities on one floor, they could consider having an extension built which will require planning permission from their local authority. It would also be wise to engage a surveyor or architect to confirm if such a major adaptation to their property is appropriate and safe.

General things

- Water heaters should be set no higher than 120^0F or 49^0C.
- Salt and other de-icing materials should be available to melt ice and snow.
- Emergency numbers should be close to a phone and names and numbers easy enough for dimming eyes to read.
- Medication should be stored where your relative can find it and dosing instructions should be included. You will need to check your relative's store of medication regularly to ensure old or out of date medication is removed. If you are concerned about them taking the correct dose, most chemists will dispense medication into blister packs, stating am/midday/pm/night time.

Home Safety Checklist

Here is a Home Safety checklist we used in a homecare service. I hope you will find it useful:

Home Safety Checklist for Older People

Crime Prevention

- Is there a good quality lock on their front and back door?

- Is there a security chain on their door?

- Does your relative know what to do when someone knocks at the door?

- Are there window locks on the ground floor?

- Has their valuable property been marked or photographed?

- Is your relative's cash kept safely in a bank or building society?

- Does your relative have a care line or personal alarm to call for help in an emergency?

Fire Safety

- Is at least one smoke detector fitted and tested regularly? Is your relative able to hear it?

- Are open fireplaces maintained, fitted with a fireguard and are chimneys swept regularly?

- Has a bedtime safety routine been explained to your relative?

- Has an escape plan in case of fire been discussed with your relative?

Falls

- Are floor surfaces non-slip and in good repair?

- Are all parts of the home well lit, including the stairs?

- Are electric cables prevented from trailing on floors in circulation areas?

- Are handrails fitted where necessary?

- Is there a bedside lamp (ideally with a motion sensor so it comes on automatically when your elderly relative moves) and torch available (in case of a power cut)?

- Do your relative's shoes and slippers fit properly and fasten securely?

- Does your relative take regular exercise?

- Is there a sturdy set of steps available to change light bulbs and reach high cupboards (your elderly relative should not do this themselves when on their own)?

- Is furniture arranged so that there is plenty of room to walk around it?

- Does your relative have a free annual eye test?

Winter Warmth

- Is your relative's home kept warm (70^0F or 20^0C)?
- Do they have at least one hot meal a day?
- Are electric blankets checked or replaced every three years?

Food Safety

- Is food fresh and does your elderly relative check "use by" dates and throw away out of date food?
- Is the fridge running at the right temperature – between 2^0C and 5^0C?

Medication

- Are medicines stored correctly according to instructions?
- Are discontinued medicines returned to the pharmacist for safe disposal?

Gas Safety

- Is gas equipment serviced regularly?
- Is there a carbon monoxide detector fitted and working?

Electrical Safety

- Are flexes checked for wear or damage?

- Are there enough sockets to avoid overloading, or multi plug adapters?

Environmental Safety

- Are there any nuisances such as noise, smells, drainage or infestations?

Water Safety

- Is the water coming from the hot water tap at hand-hot temperature and no hotter?

Equipment

There is a wide range of specialist equipment available to help older people who need help with daily living. This includes basic equipment to help with activities such as:

- Eating and drinking

- Dressing

- Going to the toilet

- Bathing

- Getting about at home

Social Services can also lend equipment to your elderly relative to enable them to:

- Use the bath
- Get on or off the toilet
- Use the stairs
- Get in or out of their home
- Remain independent if they have sensory loss

If you think that your relative needs equipment like this to manage everyday life and remain independent you need to contact their local Social Services department.

If your relative is eligible for social care support they may be able to get a Direct Payment where money is given to people with a long term illness or disability to pay for help of their choice. This can sometimes be used to purchase items of equipment.

If your relative is receiving treatment at home, their health professional, community nurse (previously called district nurse) physiotherapist or health OT can provide simple items of equipment. These include:

- Bath aids
- Trolleys
- Commodes

They may also prescribe nursing and medical equipment, such as:

- Nursing beds
- Equipment to prevent pressure sores
- Walking frames
- Crutches.

If your relative has been in hospital, the ward or Accident and Emergency Team should assess them, as part of their "going home" plan.

If you think your elderly relative needs equipment for nursing or medical care, you need to contact their GP surgery or the health professional with whom they are in contact.

Wheelchairs

If your elderly relative needs a wheelchair on a permanent basis it can be provided free of charge and maintained by their Primary Care Trust. However, they will not get a choice as to which wheelchair is provided. If they would prefer to choose their own wheelchair, they may be given an NHS voucher, which can be used to pay for it. If the voucher doesn't cover the cost of the one they want, your relative will need to make up the difference themself.

If your relative needs a wheelchair for short-term use such as a holiday, you can usually hire one from the Red Cross who do not make a charge, but ask for a donation to help them cover the cost of providing the service.

Mobility Aids

If your relative needs a walking stick or frame they should talk to their GP who can refer them to the Occupational Therapy Department at their local hospital. This is so they can be measured and given the right height walking stick or type of walking frame for them, which is important. It is therefore better to resist buying mobility aids from charity shops.

Telecare

Telecare technology is an extension of the community alarm scheme. Devices range from press-button alerts that link to a monitoring centre, to systems that aid memory or monitor well being and the environment and warn if a person's health has deteriorated. The equipment supports a person's safety and helps them to continue living independently in their own home. It can also detect dangers within the home such as smoke, flooding and gas leaks.

Telecare can also detect personal risk, such as falls and epilepsy, and a property's exit if there are concerns over someone leaving their home without support. Telecare can call for help if needed and can even remind someone to take his or her medication or turn their catheter tap off.

Environmental sensors

There are sensors that detect: extreme temperature, to prevent hypothermia; gas, if a cooker or fire has been left on/ water if a tap has been left on or there has been a leak somewhere; heat for fire safety; smoke and carbon monoxide.

Movement detectors

These can be helpful if your relative is prone to falls or experiences confusion. Sensors can detect if they are in or out of their bed or chair. Other sensors can detect whether your relative has fallen down by placing a pressure mat by their bed for example. A fall detector can also be placed on their clothes during the day.

Reminders

Voice message reminders can be used to meet a variety of needs, including asking if your relative has had their lunch, taken their medication, fed their pet or in my mother's case, remembered to turn the tap off on her catheter after she had emptied it. Mum also used a medicine dispenser that sounded an alarm to remind her to take her medication and the compartment of the medicine holder opened at the correct time of day.

Alerts for carers

If you care for your relative in your home, there are devices that sound and vibrate to alert you if for example, they leave their bed for a longer time than usual to use the bathroom. These can help you get good night's sleep because it would alert you if your relative got up at night.

There are important things for you and your relative to consider when thinking about using

Telecare, primarily the security of information it collects and whether your relative is able to give their consent. This is especially relevant if they have dementia. If they are unable to make a decision themselves, you may have to act in their best interest and make the decision for them.

Questions to ask when you are thinking about using Telecare include:

- Have your relative's views about Telecare been taken into account and do they consent to using it?
- Does your relative understand the way the equipment will work? (My parents really struggled with this.) Will having Telecare make things easier for them or will it increase their anxiety and confusion?
- Will Telecare increase their independence or lessen their ability to do things for themselves?
- Have other options been considered and is Telecare the most appropriate solution for them?

Eligibility for Telecare varies according to where you live. Some Social Services departments do not charge, taking the view that increasing older people's independence and reducing home care costs will save them money in the longer term. Others apply the same eligibility criteria across all their services, including Telecare.

John's Story

John's father, who lives alone in his flat, had recently become forgetful but made it clear that he wanted to remain in control of his life. Things came to a head when he had a fall and his son found that his father had forgotten to take his medication correctly. This happened soon after his father had left the tap on when running his bath and he became distracted when the telephone rang, causing it to overflow into the flat downstairs.

John became concerned about his father's ability to cope and worried about his safety. He wanted to make sure his father was taking his medication correctly and was keeping himself safe, so rang him several times a day to check he had taken his medication and was generally ok. The frequent calls irritated John's father and he felt under pressure to accept help that he didn't want.

Following an assessment by Social Services, John's father was happy to agree to a medicine dispenser and flood detector that would alert John if needed. His father was thus enabled to take his medication safely without having to be reminded by John and would be alerted if he left the tap on and could turn it off and avoid a flood.

Buying equipment

With an ageing population, equipment to maintain independence is big business and new ideas are being brought to the market place on a regular basis. Some of this can be expensive and I would urge you to take advice from an OT before buying large or expensive pieces of equipment. I had an aunt who had two brand new wheelchairs in her garage when she died because my uncle refused to get advice about the most suitable make and model for her.

The Government has introduced a new "retail model" which Social Services and their health partners are beginning to take up. This allows more choice and control over equipment for the people who need to use it and their carers.

In the new system, "prescriptions" are issued where there is an assessed need for equipment, which can be exchanged for free equipment at an accredited retailer. Home delivery and fitting are also funded if they are part of the assessed need. Improvements like a web-based information portal that will provide a self-assessment tool is also being developed.

The new model is intended to cover adults and carers who currently receive equipment provided by Social Services and also provide a service to people who do not choose to access public funded community equipment services as well as those who are not eligible for Social Services provision.

Descriptions for the basic equipment have been provided in a catalogue, which also contains the tariff price. If your relative wants to obtain an alternative piece of equipment that is not in the national catalogue, they will have the opportunity to "top up" the prescription.

My parents' journey continues

Equipment has played an important role in my parents' journey of increasing dependence. The NHS provided a wheelchair for my mother about ten years ago for external use. Then, as part of her initial care package and following an OT assessment, a bath hoist was installed to help her get in and out of the bath. She was also given a perch stool to use when she did the washing up and while she was washing in the bathroom and a walking frame to help her mobility. In addition, a sturdy trolley enabled Mum to transport food and drinks carefully.

Soon after my father was registered blind, he attended a rehabilitation group once a week for six weeks arranged by Social Services. In addition to a white stick he purchased a talking alarm clock and other small items to help manage his life with limited vision.

When my parents were given a Personal Budget three years later we asked Social Services for a "one-off" grant to purchase some assistive technology.

Here is what we bought at that time:

- A community care alarm was set up to enable my mother to get help in an emergency. As time went on and my father's needs increased, I got another for my father.

- A medication dispenser. The pharmacist dispensed Mum's medication into a dispenser, which was set up with an alarm to remind her to take it.

- An enuresis sensor to put in Mum's bed between the mattress cover and the sheet to detect moisture. This rang an alarm if only a drop of urine (or any other liquid) came into contact with it. This was used in the early days when Mum began forgetting to turn off the tap on her catheter, to avoid having to change and wash her bedding.
- A light over Mum's bed with a motion sensor to ensure she could see what she was doing if she got up during the night.

Points to remember

- It is important that you ensure your elderly relative's home environment is safe.
- When you are considering buying a large or expensive piece of equipment, it is important that you get advice from an occupational therapist.
- New technology, called Telecare can offer a way to detect dangers and personal risk, as well as providing aids for memory and monitoring health and well-being.

Did you know?

Older people experience more accidents in the home than younger people, often because it is not set up correctly.

8. HOMECARE MATTERS

In this chapter we will explore some of the care and support services available to provide care for your elderly relative in their own home.

Care at home (called domiciliary care or homecare) helps give independence to as many aspects of daily living as possible for people who need personal care and support at home. It can be provided by Social Services, private or voluntary organisations and can prevent the need for residential or nursing home care.

Homecare may be considered if your relative needs assistance with personal care, including getting up and going to bed, dressing, washing and personal hygiene, and preparing meals and drinks. Care workers can also offer emotional support and encouragement.

Homecare services may include support and encouragement with:

- Housework and help to do chores such as laundry and cleaning.

- Cooking, shopping, collecting prescriptions and other tasks.

- Helping someone get out and about or providing company for them while their relative goes out.

- Staying overnight.

- Help to get up in the morning, get ready for bed in the evening, and wash and bathe (personal care).

- Help to settle back home on return from a stay in hospital or help to prepare if going on holiday.

- Help with exercises recommended by a doctor, physiotherapist or other health professional.

- Support with taking medication.

Help can vary from one hour a week, to several times a day, or a live-in service in a person's home. The pattern and type of service should be designed around your relative's needs and preferences to achieve the goals set out in their care plan.

Homecare provided by a care agency

Homecare will be the first choice for elderly relatives who need help with their personal care, to lead independent lives. Typically people use a homecare service as an alternative to residential care.

The Care Quality Commission regulates care and nursing homes and also regulates homecare agencies. Regulations require that homecare workers undergo initial training to ensure they have basic knowledge and skills required for their role. Homecare workers will also have a Criminal Record Bureau (CRB) check, previously called a police check. Homecare agencies are required to comply with health and safety legislation to minimise risks to people receiving care as well as their staff.

It is important to be clear about the type of help your relative needs in order to establish whether a particular agency can meet their needs. A Social Services needs assessment can be helpful for this, even if your relative does not qualify for support from them.

You or your relative will need to discuss with the agency how their care needs can be met. For example, depending on the level of care they need, it may not be possible for one person to provide it all. A planned rota of care workers can help to minimise disruption and provide continuity.

Here are some questions to ask when you are choosing a homecare provider.

- What services do you provide?
- What are your hourly rates?
- Is it different at any time e.g. weekends?
- Are there any additional costs e.g. mileage for the carer to get to my relative's home?
- Is there a minimum time or cost my relative would be committed to?
- If my relative needs more help at short notice, would this be available?
- When do you change the prices for your service?
- How does my relative pay for the service; will you send them a bill?
- Will my relative have the same care worker come at agreed times?
- How will you match the most suitable worker to meet my relative's needs?
- How do you make sure that the person coming to help my relative knows what they need and how to support them?

- What sort of training do your care workers receive before they start work?
- What will happen when my relative's regular care worker is on holiday or off sick?
- Can care workers help with medication or with exercises my relative's GP or physiotherapist has recommended?
- What happens if my relative does not like the care worker you send; can they choose someone else?
- Can my relative contact you during the evening or at the weekend if they have a problem?

Employing your own staff

In addition to buying personal care from an agency your relative can choose to employ their own staff, called Personal Assistants (PAs), just as my parents did. Although not for everyone, there are many advantages and you, or one of their other relatives, can help them to recruit, pay and manage their PAs.

If your relative chooses to employ their own staff you should carefully consider the duties they require and write a job description so there are no misunderstandings by your relative or their staff about what is expected of them. I also drew up a profile with my parents, of the kind of person they wanted to provide their care and support. For example, my mother wanted a female over the age of twenty five, who drives and has a car to take her to appointments and be flexible with working hours and the tasks they were willing to undertake. This proved useful when we were writing the advertisement and interviewing potential staff.

Consider advertising in your relative's local newspaper and on notice boards in their local area. You should use a box number and take up references. It is also better to interview staff away from your relative's home. We booked a room in a local community centre for a couple of hours when selecting our staff.

Employing your own staff should not be taken lightly and it is important to be clear about what you are taking on. You or your relative will legally be the "the employer", a role which attracts responsibilities such as giving workers a contract of employment, working out how much tax and insurance they have to pay or how much redundancy payment staff maybe entitled to if your relative moves into a home.

Although this may sound daunting, most areas have a user led or voluntary organisation that provides support for people employing their own staff. I use one for my parents, called the Independent Living Association. They gave us templates for contracts of employment and job descriptions, provide a pay roll service and give advice about selection and recruitment, redundancy, terminating employment and other employment issues.

Of course your relative will probably need other kinds of support to help them live at home, for example with housework and gardening. If you are buying personal care and domestic help from an agency, you can sometimes purchase domestic help at a lower rate than personal care.

Live-in care

If your relative needs on-going care and support, having a live-in carer can be an excellent alternative to residential care for some people. The number of carers involved is also reduced which can provide an especially good option if your relative lives in a rural area.

The carer must have his or her own room and may need time off depending on the model of live in care your relative chooses. Don't forget to include a budget for the carer's food when thinking about the overall cost.

If your relative is eligible for funding from Social Services, you will need to check whether they will pay for a live-in carer, as it can work out higher than residential care, although not always. You also have the option of "topping-up" the funding from Social Services although this must be done by a third party as it is illegal for your relative to do this themself.

There are providers who exclusively provide live in care and these offer maximum consistency of carers. Most home care providers also offer live in care using a small team of carers who rotate to provide 24-hour care. It is important to shop around. Asking Social Services which agencies provide this service will save you time. Finally, always ask to meet the Carer with your relative before confirming the arrangement to ensure they will be compatible. You may have to see several to find the right one for your relative.

There is a wide range of services to help your relative continue living, comfortably, independently and safely in their own home. It will be helpful when you are choosing a service to know what level of support you are looking for, whether it is a little help with the housework occasionally, daily visits to help your relative get up and about, or someone living in their home full-time to be available whenever they need them.

What to do next

When you have found a suitable homecare agency, arrange an appointment for them to visit your relative. Make sure you are satisfied with everything that is being offered. It may be helpful to be with your relative when they visit to make sure that everything you need to know is covered.

As you discuss your needs with the care agency, they may suggest ways to help your relative that neither you nor your relative had considered or did not know about. It is part of the care provider's role to make things easier for your relative, which will mean that their care workers can help to look after them better.

When you choose your care agency they will provide your relative with their customer or service user pack, which will include details of what your relative has agreed with them, how you can change this and what to do if you or your relative is dissatisfied with their service. It is a legal requirement that they are given this information. The care agency will also need to check with you and your relative at least twice a year in person that you are satisfied with what you are receiving and review the service with you.

If you have recruited Personal Assistants for your relative, you will need to make sure they are aware of your expectations and identify any training needs they may have. You can find out where this training can be provided by contacting Social Services or an organisation such as PA Net www.panet.org.uk who provide information about training for PAs.

It is important to carry out a review of arrangements with PAs to discuss how they are getting on with your relative and any difficulties they may be having with the work. You also need to give them feedback on how things are working out from you and your relative's perspective.

If things are not working out you need to discuss the improvements you want to see and make a date for a further review. If their performance remains unsatisfactory, you will need to give them notice and I suggest you contact PA Net (see above) who offer employment information and advice to those who employ PAs.

Whether your relative uses an agency or employs their own care workers you will find completing and sharing the following checklist helpful for informing staff about your relative's needs.

Essential Information Checklist

Name _____

Likes to be called _____

Next of kin/emergency contact details_____

_____

_____

GP details _____

_____

_____

Key safe number _____

Medical conditions _____

_____

_____

_____

Medication _____

_____

_____

_____

Is/Is not living with dementia

If yes, severity:

☐ Mild

☐ Moderate

☐ Severe

Orientation:

☐ Verbal or visual prompts

☐ Requires orientation to time, person and place

☐ Observation as may try to leave unsupported

Anxiety and distress

☐ Emotionally anxious

☐ Verbal aggression

☐ Physical aggression

☐ Triggers

☐ Support required

Mobility

☐ Wheelchair

☐ Frame

☐ Walking stick

☐ Needs physical assistance

☐ History of falls

Continence

- [ ] Fully independent
- [ ] Requires reminders
- [ ] Catheter
- [ ] Incontinent of urine
- [ ] Incontinent of faeces
- [ ] Double incontinence
- [ ] Uses pads for confidence
- [ ] Assistance of one carer
- [ ] Assistance of two carers
- [ ] Hoist

Communication

- [ ] Blind or partially sighted
- [ ] Hearing impairment
- [ ] Language

Dietary requirements

- [ ] Diabetic
- [ ] Cultural
- [ ] Preferences
- [ ] Low fat
- [ ] Swallowing/choking issues
- [ ] Softened diet
- [ ] Thickened fluids
- [ ] Hobbies/Interests

Emma's Story

Emma had been concerned about her mother Martha for a while, because she had been showing signs of dementia, such as repeating questions to Emma and becoming confused when she carried out basic tasks like preparing scrambled eggs or heating a pizza. Eventually Martha was diagnosed with Alzheimer's disease, the most common form of dementia.

At first Emma and her sister took turns staying with their mother but soon found they could not keep it up. They found a small day centre not far away, which specialised in looking after people with dementia, so Emma arranged for her mother to attend, five days a week. This enabled Emma to continue her career as a physiotherapist and her sister to spend more time looking after her husband, who recently had a stroke. When Martha attended the day centre, Emma and her sister knew their mother was safe, socially stimulated and receiving nourishing food and regular drinks.

As her mother's disease progressed over the next few years, Emma arranged for regular carers from an agency to provide care and support for her mother before and after she attended the day centre as well as during the evening and at weekends.

To help provide consistency, Emma was advised to set up a care journal for her mother. Whoever was with Martha, would record the important details of their shift, such as food eaten, fluids consumed, bowel and bladder movements, activities accomplished and other relevant information.

Emma, her sister and the care workers became proficient at using the hospital bed and hoist provided by the district nurse, a wheelchair, wheelchair ramps and a food processor to prepare easy to chew, soft food as Martha had chosen not to wear her dentures. Emma arranged for *Meals on Wheels* to be delivered on a Saturday to give her a break from preparing food and free up time to take her mother out.

When her mother became ill with pneumonia, Emma took special leave from work and moved in to look after her. During Martha's last forty-eight hours of life, she was loved and comforted by Emma and her sister, attended by the district nurse and heard her son's voice over the phone, all the way from Australia.

Meals

A *Meals on Wheels* service is available to anyone who cannot get to the shop, is unwell, or unable to prepare and cook a meal. They can also be delivered if a carer or relative is having a break, away on holiday or is ill. Meals can be ordered by the person themself, relatives or friends.

Social Service departments all have their own arrangements for providing *Meals on Wheels*. In most areas the *Women's Royal Voluntary Service* (WRVS), *Age UK* or other voluntary organisation runs the scheme.

Hot and frozen meals are usually available and provided at a subsidised rate for people who are eligible for social care funding. Frozen meals will enable your relative to decide what they want to eat on a daily basis as well as the time they want to eat. The meals can usually be heated in a microwave, which is safer than an oven. On the other hand having a hot meal delivered every day ensures your relative is having a nutritious meal each day and provides someone to check your relative is up and about. If the person delivering the meal doesn't get a reply they will report the matter, which will be checked out.

There is also a plethora of private organisations offering frozen and occasionally hot meals. You can find out which ones deliver in your relative's area by contacting their local Social Services or looking in the telephone directory. Some people also use the many varieties of ready meals available from supermarkets.

Fresh vegetables and home cooked food have always been a priority in my family. My mother had to give up cooking when her memory began to deteriorate over twenty years ago and my father was an excellent cook until his memory also failed more recently. We have tried at least four private companies as well as *Meals on Wheels* and after a while my parents find a problem with them. We are currently using a mix of ready meals from *M&S*, an excellent company called *Cook* and meals that I have cooked myself and frozen for them.

Ensuring my parents have a balanced and nutritional diet is increasingly challenging, as my father frequently feels too tired or forgets to prepare meals – even basic things like scrambled eggs. I am also finding it difficult to ensure they have their "five-a-day" fruit and vegetables. This role reversal feels strange, as it doesn't seem long ago that my parents were nagging me to "Eat your veggies".

Day Centres

Day services not only help people to maintain independence, but they can give carers and relatives a break from their caring role. Services are often provided from a dedicated day centre or sometimes a care home. They can include:

- Specialist support for people with complex needs.
- Assistance with personal care, such as bathing.
- Rehabilitation to help regain, improve or maintain living skills and mobility.
- Building links with community activities and clubs.
- The opportunity to mix with other people and participate in social activities, including hobbies and interests.
- A main meal and refreshments.
- Support with arrangements for transport to and from the service.

Day activities and clubs

A range of activities takes place within the local community, which are available for older people. These can include special interest groups, volunteering opportunities and education classes.

There are also luncheon clubs, often run by voluntary organisations such as *Age UK* or maybe linked to local churches or communities.

Arranging services

Whenever I am supporting someone to arrange for a tradesman to attend to something in their home or garden, I always check the directory offered by most Trading Standards departments called "Buying with Confidence". Every trader and business listed in this guide has been vetted by Trading Standards officers to ensure that they:

- Are committed to fair trading and to providing a quality service for their customers.
- Can produce Criminal Records Bureau checks for staff who want to work in people's homes.
- Make sure their staff are competent for the work they carry out.
- Deal with customers promptly, efficiently and courteously.
- Undertake to comply with the spirit of the letter of the law and not restrict customers' rights.
- Have a sound customer complaints procedure.

Points to remember

- Homecare can be provided by a care agency or by your relative employing their own staff.

- You need to be clear about the type of help your relative needs when considering whether a particular agency can meet their needs.

- Balanced and nutritious meals are important for your relative. If they are unable to prepare and cook a meal themselves, meals can be provided by Social Services' *Meals on Wheels* service, a private company, or by purchasing frozen meals from a supermarket.

- Day centres can provide a number of important functions including helping people maintain their independence and giving relatives and carers a break.

Did you know?

Four out of every five older people in the UK needing care, arrange to receive support in their own home.

9. RESIDENTIAL MATTERS

In this chapter we will re-join my parents' journey, look at the different types of residential care and consider what to look for when choosing a care or nursing home.

My parents have become more dependent on me and my father's health has deteriorated significantly. They have begun arguing a lot, which is probably due to their increasing frustration and fear about their diminishing independence. Just before Christmas my father told me that he was no longer able to cope with looking after my mother and asked if the family could get together when my brother and I returned from holiday in the new year to discuss options.

Even though I could see it coming, hearing Dad say that he could no longer cope with Mum was a shock and my heart sank as I began thinking about the inevitable outcome that I knew would break my mother's heart. Mum would have to move into a care home and, after sixty-four years together, they would be separated. Moreover, Mum had always maintained that she would take her own life if my father died before her and I feared she would consider moving away from my father in a similar way. I was overcome by a deep sense of guilt and felt that, despite all my knowledge and experience, I could not come up with a viable alternative to residential care and had therefore let Mum down.

Christmas came and went with a cloud hanging over my brother, sister and me. We spent hours talking about different options to keep Mum and Dad living together. Dad would not meet the criteria for Social Services to enable him to go into a care home with her and did not feel ready to give up his independence anyway.

The only possible alternative to residential care would be to have a live in carer but my parents only have two bedrooms and Mum and Dad had one each. We thought about turning their lounge into a bed-sit for Mum to free up a room for the carer and got excited about this idea for a while. However, by the time we got together for the family meeting, it had became apparent that Mum's obsessive dependence on Dad and the mental pressure she exerted on him, ruled this out as a viable option. Even with the practical help from a carer, Mum would be unable to leave Dad alone when she needed reassurance, which was most of the time. Dad just could not cope with this any longer.

Before telling my mother that she would need to move into a care home, we agreed that my brother and I would look for suitable care homes. My sister lives over fifty miles away so it wasn't practical for her to help us with the initial search. We drew up a short list of the things that would be important for Mum. The home had to:

- Accept the level of funding that Social Services would pay.

- Be less than fifteen minutes travelling distance from my father, as he is unable to sit in a car for longer.

- Have en-suite facilities (we knew that Mum would be really anxious about sharing a loo).

- Have level access or a lift (neither Mum nor Dad is able to manage steps or stairs).

- Have a non-clinical, homely atmosphere.

- Have a good report from the regulatory body.

I looked at more than twenty homes and my brother joined me for some of the visits (he works shifts so was not always able to join me).We short-listed three for Mum to have a look at that met our criteria and had a vacancy. I found looking around homes time consuming and was grateful for my knowledge of the local care home market, without which the task would have taken even longer.

I knew how devastated Mum would be at having to leave my father and was relieved when their GP offered to break the news to her about having to go into a home. My sister and brother-in-law arranged to visit the following week to take Mum to look at the homes, while I stayed home with my father, who was unwell at the time.

When they returned I was told Mum had looked around the homes in a disinterested manner except for one room in one of the homes. It was number seventeen, which was the number of her childhood home, and the colour scheme was mauve, her favourite colour. Although Mum remained resigned and apathetic, these factors were the best indication that she had made a choice as it was the only room in which she had shown any interest whatsoever.

I let Social Services know which care home Mum had chosen and a social worker visited the home to negotiate the fees, make sure it was able to meet Mum's needs and sign the contract. The manager of the home also came and assessed her, to make sure the home would be able to meet her needs. We arranged the date Mum would move into the home and confirmed that it would be for a month's trial to see if she liked it.

The move was traumatic for Mum and Dad who were equally devastated. Dad felt guilty at not being able to look after his wife and was like a fish out of water. His days had been totally structured around Mum and he was disorientated on his own. I made out a daily and weekly routine for him in large print, which seemed to help, and visited him more often to check that he was looking after himself.

If your relative is thinking of moving to a care home, they will be faced with some important decisions and choices. They will need information about the options available to them and guidance about the questions they may wish to ask. The information available in this chapter will help you to both gather information and ask the right questions before making your choice.

The decision to leave their home and move into a care home is not an easy one. They may be thinking about it because they are finding it difficult to cope, perhaps they are becoming frail and need help. It may be that the primary carer is no longer able to cope, like my father. Wherever possible, care and support services will be available to help them continue to live at home. In some cases, however, it may be that residential or nursing home care is the right option for them.

There are three main types of care home:

Care home (residential)

A residential care home provides the care and support your relative would receive at home from a carer. Staff can help with personal care such as washing, taking a bath or shower, getting up, dressing and assistance with eating and drinking.

Help is available twenty-four hours a day and meals are provided, usually with a choice of main meal. Activities and outings are usually available and visitors are always welcome. Care homes aim to help people lead an independent life in as homely a setting as possible.

Long-term care fees are expensive and as soon as you are starting to think about residential care I strongly advise you to seek specialist financial advice. You can find information about this in the section 'specialist financial advice about long-term-care' in Chapter 12.

Care Home (special needs)

Specialist care homes, which used to be called EMI (Elderly Mentally Infirm) homes, are care homes registered for people with dementia. The particular needs of people with dementia mean more staff are required who receive training to help them manage the problematic behaviour associated with Alzheimer's and other forms of dementia.

Care homes (nursing)

Care homes with nursing generally care for more dependent people who have more complex and/or changing care needs and require the sort of care that can only be provided under the supervision of a qualified nurse. Accordingly they are required by law to have a qualified nurse on duty twenty-four hours a day.

Some care homes provide both residential and nursing care and are sometimes referred to as dual registered homes. You may decide to choose a home like this so your elderly relative doesn't need to move again if their needs change.

If your relative needs residential or nursing care and Social Services have agreed to give them financial help, they can still choose where they want to live. The home may be provided by Social Services or be run independently, but it must be a home that:

- Has been approved by Social Services.
- Is suitable for your relative's assessed needs.
- Will enter into a contract with Social Services.
- Has a vacancy.

- Is within their financial limit of support for your relative's assessed level of need.

If you and your relative choose a home which costs more than Social Services are willing to pay for, you or any other third party can pay the difference. However it is illegal for your relative to top up their own funding.

You may make your own arrangements to choose a home your relative prefers and they can pay the cost themselves. This could be because your relative needs care in a residential or nursing home but they are not eligible to receive financial help from Social Services. If your relative doesn't need care in a residential or nursing home, they may still choose to go into an independent home and pay the full cost themselves. If choosing this option, I would advise you get independent financial advice about funding long-term care to help you make the right choices.

When you are beginning to think about a care home for your elderly relative, you need to consider the area in which it would be best for them to live. Would they like to live near you or other relatives? Would that take them away from their friends and neighbours? Remember, even if Social Services have agreed to contribute towards funding, your relative can still move to another area if they want to, but think about it carefully first.

Once you and your relative have decided where they would like to live, the next step is to think about what type of home your relative needs. The assessment carried out on your relative will have determined whether they need a nursing home, residential care home or a specialist home such as one for people with dementia. Next you need to find out what homes there are in the area in which they have chosen to live. To find this out, contact the Social Services department responsible for that area and ask them to send you a list of approved residential care and nursing homes.

Having determined which category of care home your relative needs, make a short list of those that match your criteria. You will only find out about some of the things on your list by phoning the home and asking.

Social workers are not allowed to make recommendations and if your elderly relative is not eligible for financial help from Social Services you will have to find a suitable care or nursing home yourselves. The selection process can take time and be difficult. If your relative is eligible for funding from Social Services you can ask for a social worker to help you. If not you might find it helpful to get a professional such as an independent care consultant to help you. They can save you time and also negotiate fees on your relative's behalf, which can sometimes save money towards the cost of their fees.

Once you have found out about the homes in the area in which your relative wants to live, the next thing to do is make a list of the things that are important to them. Make an appointment with the homes you want to look around and take the list with you when you visit them. You will find there are a lot of other things to consider. Don't worry about asking too many questions when you look round a home. It is sensible to do as much research as possible when you are making such a life changing decision. If you are able to, speak to some of the residents at the home, they will be able to give you a realistic view about what it is like to live there.

When going into a care or nursing home use your eyes and nose. First impressions really do count and if the home doesn't smell pleasant then you are probably in the wrong place for your relative. Look at the décor. Is the home well maintained? Look at the people. Are the staff smiling and interacting with residents and more importantly, are the residents smiling and engaged in what is happening around them?

Questions to ask when considering a care home for your relative

- In what circumstances would your relative be asked to leave and what would happen if they run out of funds?
- How does the home handle complaints? Is there a residents' committee and a relatives' group?
- What would happen if your relative becomes ill and needs more care, would they have to move?
- Will your relative be offered a choice of meals and can they choose when and where they eat?
- Does the room have an en-suite bathroom? Is it suitable to meet your relative's needs?
- Is there a TV and telephone point in the room?
- What is the ratio of staff to residents? How many staff are on duty at night?
- Are shops and library within walking distance?
- Does the home offer activities and an entertainment programme?
- Is there a garden?
- Can your relative keep their GP and manage their own medication if they want to?
- Does the home allow pets?

- Will your relative be able to choose when they get up and go to bed?
- Can your relative choose to have some meals in their room?

It is important to check with a home whether they are able to meet your relative's specific care needs such as dementia or incontinence and how they manage the progression of these and other conditions. If your relative has a condition that is likely to deteriorate, ask what will happen if they need to be moved.

Finally, ask for a copy of the care home's most recent inspection report and a copy of their Statement of Purpose. This sets out their aims and objectives and the services and facilities they offer.

When you have finished you need to ask the most important question of all. Would I like to live in this home myself? Keep looking if the answer is no!

Once you and your relative have decided which home is best for them, the manager or matron of the home will want to carry out an assessment to ensure they can meet your relative's care needs before they will accept them.

The first four weeks of their stay will be a trial period as it is never possible to be completely sure that your relative will like the home. The trial period gives your relative time to get used to the home and see if it can meet their needs. You may feel that another home might be more suitable, or your relative may wish to return home with a care package to support them.

Ella's Story

Ella's seventy year-old aunt, Kate, was admitted to a nursing home after a prolonged spell in hospital, which was fully funded by Continuing Healthcare. She suffered from a number of chronic health problems and had been recently diagnosed with a condition that resulted in a high risk of her choking.

Kate frequently lamented to Ella that she hated being in the nursing home and desperately wanted to return to her own home. Health professionals felt the risk of her choking to death was too high for Kate to be cared for in a domestic setting but Ella wanted to support her aunt to go home if at all possible.

Ella was advised that a joint health and social care Risk Enablement Panel was held in her area every week. She made contact with the person who chaired the panel and asked for her aunt's case to be included on the agenda. This was done and three weeks later Ella was invited to present her aunt's case to the panel.

Having been fully briefed beforehand, Ella set out her aunt's case to return home and the lead health professional set out his case for Kate to remain in a health setting. Elle left her trump card until the end as she had been advised to do. This was that Ella had undertaken a study of the contact time Kate had with staff and found that for more than seventy percent of the time, her aunt was unsupervised and on her own. This contrasted with only sixty-two percent unsupervised time with the proposed intensive care package. With the addition of Telecare equipment, her chosen option offered higher mitigation against Kate's risk of choking. Ella also made the point that her aunt had a right to choose where she lived and died. If Kate did end up choking to death, she wanted to do it in her own home.

Following detailed planning, training for the team of agency care workers, guidelines about action to be taken in the event of Kate choking (written by a speech and language therapist, trained to manage problems with swallowing) and installation of Telecare equipment, Kate returned home six weeks later.

The Role of the Care Quality Commission (CQC)

All homecare services, care and nursing homes, NHS and private hospitals and GP practices, must be registered with the Care Quality Commission (CQC), an independent government body that is responsible for the regulation of community or integrated healthcare, community social care, care and nursing homes and rehabilitation services.

The Commission carries out inspections of all care homes and home care providers to ensure they meet essential standards of quality and safety. Inspection reports on each home and homecare provider are available from CQC or the care home or organisation itself and these should be taken into account when making a decision.

Where an inspection highlights outcomes that do not meet the essential standards, the service is given a period of time in which to address those issues. If they fail to do so, the CQC can take enforcement action, which could result in cancellation of registration.

The way the CQC carry out inspections is changing against a backdrop of scandalous failures in the care system. In April 2013 the CQC launched a new strategy, to make sure health and social care services provide people with safe, effective, compassionate, high-quality care and to encourage care services to improve.

To achieve this, they are acting on the recommendations of the report into the abuse of people with learning disabilities at Winterbourne View, Robert Francis' report into the failings at Mid Staffordshire NHS Foundation Trust and the government's response to catastrophic failures of care in Patients First and Foremost.

The changes will be implemented following extensive consultation and some will take up to three years to make.

The CQC plan is to inspect and regulate different services in different ways based on what has the most impact on the quality of people's care. However, there are fundamental principles that will guide their work:

When they carry out an inspection they will ask the following questions about care services:

- Are they safe?
- Are they effective?
- Are they caring?
- Are they responsive to people's needs?
- Are they well led?

Points to remember

- There are three main types of care home. One provides the care and support your relative would receive in their own home. Another provides twenty-four hour care for people with special needs such as dementia. The third provides residential care with nursing care and support under the supervision of a qualified nurse, twenty-four hours a day.

- Choosing the right care home for your elderly relative is important because it will be a life changing experience for them and like everything else, there are good and bad homes.

- Care and nursing homes are regulated by the Care Quality Commission (CQC) who carry out inspections of all care homes to ensure they meet essential standards of quality and safety.

- The first four weeks after admission will be a trial period for your relative to see if they like the home and ensure it is the right one for them.

Did you know?

Over thirty percent of people who fund their own care, only visit one care or nursing home prior to admission.

10. RESIDENTIAL LIVING MATTERS

In this chapter we will catch up with how my mother is settling into her care home and consider the issues that are likely to affect your elderly relative when they move into a residential setting.

Getting Mum settled into the home has been a huge challenge and we are not there yet. Without a doubt she did not want to go into a home and is a victim of circumstance in that she needs a lot of looking after and Dad is no longer able to do this. I never thought Mum would have to go into a home and would have given anything to keep her at home with my father.

The days and weeks after Mum went into the care home were difficult. She vacillated between tearful depression, angry outbursts and belligerent behaviour. A couple of times she made half-hearted attempts on her life to let us all know how much she was hurting. Dad was like a fish out of water and I found that nothing in my professional training and vast experience of working with older people and their families had prepared me for the emotional roller coaster upon which I found myself.

It is always difficult when there are mental health issues as well as chronic physical conditions. Mum suffers from dementia as well as severe anxiety and depression, which can be very wearing for anyone looking after her. She constantly needs reassurance and became so demanding and dependent on my father that he just couldn't cope anymore. Indeed, their GP, who is a great doctor in my opinion, told us that Dad had continued looking after my mother far longer than would most other people.

In common with many older people, my mother has an unrealistic perception of her abilities and thinks she can do much more for herself than she can. She also has no awareness whatsoever of the effect her mental state has on other people, especially my father. As a result she is unable to understand why she had to move into a care home and believes it is because my father and the rest of us no longer love her. This is so very far from the truth.

In my experience, people often think that they can do more than they can when they grow older and it makes me think about something my mother said to me years ago: "The hardest thing about growing older is that you still feel young inside". As I grow older myself, I know just how true this is.

You may wonder why I didn't have my mother live with me. The answer is that I was still working full-time and I live in a flat. Moreover, I know that it could have destroyed our relationship, as I have seen many loving relationships turn into resentment and bitterness when an elderly relative – especially one with mental health problems – moves in. Far better, I thought, to have other people look after Mum on a day-to-day basis, leaving the family to show our love by visiting as often as we can and taking her out regularly.

The manager and staff at the home have been wonderful with Mum since she moved in and I believe our research paid off. I had a telephone installed in her room, although this has sometimes caused a problem when she phones and leaves messages telling us how unhappy she is. I keep in regular contact with the manager who reassures me that Mum is fine the rest of the time. I believe this is true because on one occasion when Mum didn't know I was standing behind the door, she was laughing and joking with a member of staff, but when she saw me she burst into tears and told me how unhappy she was. When I was training to be a Social Worker I remember reading a well-known book by a psychologist, Eric Byrne called *The Games People Play*. I think my next book will be called "The Games Mothers Play".

Important issues when moving into a care home

Contract and fees

Once you have found a suitable care or nursing home, you need to check that the fees and contract terms are acceptable – both to your relative and to Social Services if they are contributing to the cost. If your relative is funding their own care, they should be given a written contract. If Social Services are helping with the cost, they will produce the contract but your relative should receive a copy of the home's terms and conditions.

The contract, or terms and conditions, should be clear and include the following:

- The fees, what is included and what is extra.
- Whether fees are payable in advance.
- How any contribution from Social Services and/or the NHS towards the cost is handled.

- What notice is required before leaving.
- How temporary absences such as visits to stay with family or hospital stays are charged for.
- Any charges that may be made after a person's death.

The contract should be clear without you needing to take legal advice, stating clearly the date from when fees are due and the period fees are charged. There are usually services that are not included in the fees so check what your relative is paying for. The following are examples of items and services for which your relative may have to pay extra:

- Chiropody
- Dentistry
- Optician and glasses
- Hairdressing
- Telephone calls
- Dry cleaning
- Incontinence products
- Toiletries
- Travel and escort costs
- Newspapers and magazines

If you are signing a contract on behalf of your relative, you need to make sure it is clear in what capacity you are signing it. Are you taking on personal liability for the fees? Or will you be signing as an appointee or as your relative's Power of Attorney?

I believe the following issues are as important today as they were many years ago when I was responsible for managing care homes for older people (including specialist homes for people who had dementia and for older people who were blind or partially sighted).

Privacy

Moving into a residential setting can feel intrusive and life may feel more "public" as a result. For example, staff discussing one resident in front of another. Sometimes it is not so much about what people say as what they do, for example leaving the door open when helping someone with their personal care. Mum likes the door of her room kept open to see what is going on and to avoid feeling lonely and isolated, but likes it closed when we visit her. It all comes down to respecting the dignity of people and treating them as individuals.

Choice

Residents should be assisted to make choices about the things that matter to them and these should be recorded in their care plan. This should be routinely updated as people often change their mind.

Some examples are:

- Asking people what they like to be called.
- What they would like to wear.
- How they like to spend their time.

It is important that you make sure staff are aware of the things that are important to your elderly relative before they move into a care or nursing home. For example, Mum is shy and needs time to get to know people. She also, hates bingo and other games, but enjoys a good quiz.

Food and drink

A balanced and nutritious diet with plenty of fluids is an essential part of healthy residential living. Your relative should be given a choice for all meals and within reason be able to choose where they eat. For example, Mum enjoys breakfast and supper in her room. Her home does not offer a cooked breakfast and when she told me that she missed "a nice bit of bacon" I had a word with the manager and asked if she could be offered egg and bacon sometimes for supper. Mum also enjoys a glass of wine with her main meal and sometimes in the evening as well, so we take in a bottle of her favourite wine when we visit and leave it with staff to give her.

Continence

The majority of older people have difficulty in getting to and using the toilet, and the way this is managed in the home is critical. Most of us have visited someone in hospital or a care or nursing home and experienced an unpleasant smell. I avoided these places like the plague when I was looking for a care home for Mum as I believe the way continence is managed to be an indicator of the quality of care offered by the home generally. Mum has a catheter because she used to regularly suffer from urine infections. How the home could help manage her catheter was something I went through carefully with the Manager before Mum went to live in the home.

Clothing

We express our individuality by the clothes we wear and this is no different when we become older and live in a care or nursing home. Mum is very fussy that she wears clothes that match or complement each other and is able to express this to staff. However, not everyone is able to do this so be sure to make staff aware of the way your relative likes to dress.

National Care Standards

In 2010, a law was introduced for regulating healthcare and adult social care. This ensures that every care service in England is legally responsible for meeting essential standards of quality and safety.

The Care Quality Commission registers care services to ensure they meet these standards and monitors them to make sure they continue to do so. They have available a wide range of actions and penalties if they find care services are not meeting the essential standards.

The following is a summary of the essential standards that you can expect from a registered care service for your elderly relative, which is taken from the Care Quality Commission's website.

1. **You can expect to be involved and told what's happening at every stage of your care.**

- You will always be involved in discussions about your care and treatment, and all staff will respect your privacy and dignity.
- You will be given opportunities, encouragement and support to promote your independence.
- You will be able to agree or reject any type of examination, care, and treatment or support before you receive it.

2. **You can expect care, treatment and support that meets your needs.**

- Your personal needs will be assessed to make sure you get the care that is safe and supports your rights.
- You will get the food and drink you need to meet your dietary need.
- You get the treatment that you and your health or care professional agree will make a difference to your health and well-being.
- You will get safe and co-ordinated care where more than one provider is involved or if you move between services.

3. You can expect to be safe.

- You will be protected from abuse or the risk of abuse, and staff will respect your human rights.

- You will be cared for in a clean environment where you are protected from infection.

- You will get the medicines you need, when you need them, and in a safe way.

- You will be cared for in a safe and accessible place that will help you as you recover.

- You will not be harmed by unsafe or unsuitable equipment.

4. You can expect to be cared for by qualified staff.

- Your health and welfare needs are met by staff who are properly qualified.

- There will always be enough members of staff available to keep you safe and meet your health and welfare needs.

- You will be looked after by staff who are well managed and have the chance to develop and improve their skills.

5. You can expect your care provider to constantly check the quality of its services.

- Your care provider will continuously monitor the quality of its services to make sure you are safe.

- If you, or someone acting on your behalf makes a complaint, you will be listened to and it will be acted upon properly.

- Your personal records, including medical records, will be accurate and kept safe and confidential.

Lorna's Story

Whenever Lorna visited her elderly aunt who was in a care home she had to wait a long time before a member of staff opened the door to let her in. She was also concerned about the length of time it took staff to answer emergency call bells and was told by her aunt that sometimes she had an "accident" because staff took so long to help her to the toilet. When Lorna had a word about this she was told by the manager that the new owner would not let her cover staff who were off sick or on holiday. Lorna sent a written complaint to the care homeowner and copied in the Care Quality Commission. The staffing level was subsequently increased.

Points to remember

- If Social Services are not contributing to some or all of the cost, make sure you check the contract between your relative and the care home.

- If you are signing the contract on behalf of your relative, make sure that the capacity in which you are signing is clear.

- The essential standards that you can expect from a registered care service are monitored by the Care Quality Commission (CQC)

Did you know?

The average length of stay in a care home for someone funding his or her own care is 28 months.

11. CARING MATTERS

In this chapter we will consider the services available to carers, the benefits of having a carer's assessment, the circumstances that enable you to have an assessment, respite care and long-distance caring.

Carers are often family members. They are people who provide care without pay, out of love, respect, responsibility, duty etc. and can include:

- Caring for a spouse
- Caring for an elderly parent
- Caring for a sibling
- Caring for extended family
- Caring for a grandparent
- Caring for an elderly aunt or uncle

I have met many people over the years who refuse to wear the label of carer, preferring to see himself or herself as a son, daughter or other family member. For some people this is really important and their wishes should be respected. There are benefits though in using the term carer, if you provide regular care and support to someone (your relationship to them doesn't matter) because it will enable you to get help when you need it.

Social Services and NHS Trusts are given grants from central government to provide services for those carers, who provide substantial and regular support to people receiving social care support. Those services include, for example, breaks from caring responsibilities and gym and swimming fees to promote their own health and well-being. However, it is very much a postcode lottery and the priority given to providing support for carers of people who fund their own services varies enormously across the country.

The contribution that carers make is often forgotten and taken for granted. Services can be difficult to access, complicated to understand and information about available services can sometimes be difficult to obtain.

Services for Carers

Most areas will have a Carers Centre provided by a voluntary or not-for-profit organisation, which can be found by contacting Social Services in your relative's local area. Each centre provides a wide range of local support services to meet the needs of carers in their local community. This will include information about health issues, respite care services, entitlements, mobility, grants for holidays and equipment, whether or not carers receive support from Social Services.

Carer's Assessments

If you provide care and support for a substantial amount of time on a regular basis, you have a right to a carer's assessment. This has to take into account the impact caring is having on your life. A carer's assessment means Social Services will look at your situation and see if you are entitled to any services that could make caring easier for you. It is your chance to discuss with Social Services what help you need. You can also discuss help that may be available to maintain your own heath and enable you to balance caring with other areas of your life such as family, work or leisure time.

New Rights for Carers

New rights for carers were included in the Care Bill, which was published on the 10th May 2013. These, for the first time, give carers the same rights to assessments and care services from local authorities as those they care for.

However how this is to be funded and implemented has yet to be decided.

Ann's Story

Ann had been looking after her mother-in-law who has Multiple Sclerosis for nearly a year. She called in on her way to work to get her breakfast before her carers arrived and again on her way home to prepare her mother-in-law's tea. Over the weekend Ann and her husband got her shopping and provided home cooked meals. They also provide emergency cover during the night and at the weekend.

I suggested that Ann contact Social Services to ask for a carer's assessment, so she and her husband could book a holiday. Her mother's social worker told Ann that she did not qualify for a carer's assessment because she was working. I was able to reassure Ann that she was entitled to an assessment even though she was combining caring with part-time work Ann eventually got the assessment she needed.

Unfortunately some professionals are not aware of a carer's right to an assessment and some people are told incorrectly that they are not entitled to one. If this happens to you, put your request for an assessment in writing and ask why you are being refused.

As a carer you have the right to have your needs assessed separately from the person you care for. You can request an assessment if you provide regular and substantial levels of care and support, whether the person you care for lives with you or not. Carers can have an assessment even if the person they care for declines an assessment or the provision of services.

You are entitled to an assessment of your own needs even if you are living a distance away from your relative, or if the person you are caring for has not been assessed or is not receiving any services. You also have a right to an assessment if you intend to look after a relative when they return home from a period in hospital. However, you will not be eligible for an assessment unless your relative is eligible for funded social care.

Respite Care

If you, or one of the other members of your family are providing "regular and substantial care" for a relative you are entitled to a break from caring, even if support is also provided by Social Services.

Respite care means temporary relief and usually consists of extra services provided for a limited period of time to allow you to take break from your caring responsibilities. It may be provided for your elderly relative or for you. It may be for as little as an hour, a night, a day or a week or two, depending on you and your relative's circumstances.

Respite care can be provided on a regular basis or at a time of crisis, for example if you had to go into hospital. It can be provided in your relative's home, for example by having a temporary carer from an agency (who can live in if required) while you are away, or your relative may move temporarily into a care home or hospital environment.

If Social Services provide a care package for your relative, they will arrange and pay for respite breaks. If your relative has a medical need for NHS respite care the NHS will arrange and pay for respite care.

For people who fund their own services or, like my parents, have a Personal Budget from Social Services, there are other options. For example, staying together in a small hotel with a care worker from an agency visiting to provide personal care and help with dressing, or finding a home that offers respite breaks for ex-servicemen. These are merely examples. The key is to find out what is really important to your relative and plan around that.

Whether Social Services, the NHS or your relative are responsible for funding respite care, if you are providing regular care and support to your relative, it is important that you look after yourself by ensuring that you have regular breaks from caring.

Joan's Story

Joan had been caring for her husband John, for a number of years but was finding it difficult to cope, as his care needs increased.

As the couple had savings and investments they were not entitled to funding from Social Services. After talking to them both to find out which support would best meet their needs, I arranged for a care worker to sit with John twice a week while Joan went shopping or to see her friend who had been ill or to have her hair done. I also found a care home that had a good day-centre attached which John agreed to go to once a week. He enjoyed going to the centre and Joan found the Manager very supportive and knowledgeable about how to manage her husband when he became frustrated.

I also arranged for John to spend a week in the care home while Joan went away with her friend on holiday.

Caring from a Distance

If you live more than an hour or so from your elderly relative who needs care and support, you can think of yourself as a long-distance carer. This can take many forms, from money management to arranging for home care support, from providing respite care for their primary carer to creating a plan in case of emergencies. Many long distance carers act as information coordinators, helping their elderly relative understand the confusing maze of resources, including care and support options, equipment to maintain their independence, benefit claims, medical equipment and access to NHS or social care funding.

Caring, no matter where the carer lives, is often long lasting and ever expanding. For the long-distance carer, what may begin as an occasional social phone call to share family news, can eventually turn into regular phone calls about health symptoms, arranging for groceries to be delivered and managing household bills. What starts as a monthly trip to "check on Mum" may become a bigger project to move her to a care home nearer to where you live.

If you are a long-distance carer, you are not alone. Families are more disparate nowadays and move around to gain employment among other reasons.

Sometimes this takes them abroad and I know of several families where parents and their adult children all live in different countries.

Sometimes your relative may ask for help; at the sudden start of an illness for example. However when you live far away, some detective work might be necessary to uncover the signs that they need more help.

It can be difficult to know when your elderly relative needs help from phone calls, as many older people are fiercely independent and often overestimate their abilities. If you are personally unable to visit to do the detective work, you could ask another relative, friend or neighbour to pay a visit on your behalf. You need to handle the situation sensitively as your relative might not want to admit that they are often too tired to cook an entire meal. However if you visit at the time they usually have their main meal, and ask "What's cooking?" you may get a sense that dinner is a bowl of cereal and be able to offer some help. With your relative's permission, you might contact people who see your relative regularly – local relatives, friends, neighbours or a doctor for example – and ask them to drop you an email if they are concerned.

When you spend a longer visit, you can look for possible problem areas. It's easier for your relative to disguise problems during a short phone call than during a longer personal visit. You can also make the most of your visit if you take time in advance to develop a list of potential problem areas you want to check out while you are there. Of course it may not be possible to do everything in one trip, but you can prioritise potentially dangerous situations and take care of those as soon as possible, then see afterwards if you can arrange for someone else to take care of the rest. As well as safety issues, try and determine your relative's mood and general health. It is possible to confuse depression in older people (something that is under diagnosed) with normal ageing. If your relative is depressed, they may brighten up during your phone call, but find their cheerful mood difficult to maintain during a longer visit.

Staying in contact with your relative by phone or email might take the pressure off your sister who lives locally. With so much information available on the internet, long-distance carers can also play a part in arranging professional carers or carrying out first stage research to find a suitable service, such as a care home for your elderly relative. Some long distance carers I know, find they can be helpful by handling things on line, such as paying bills, researching health problems or medicines and keeping family and friends updated.

A resource I found that is particularly helpful for long distance carers is *Care Central* (www.carecentral.com). This is a website where you can create your own private, central hub to keep in touch, stay informed and share support. Only family and others that you invite will have access to your *Care Central* site. It even has a "Lend a Hand" section where you can ask for help with a specific task and members of your family can volunteer to help you.

Being a carer is not easy for anyone and both the carer and the person being cared for have to make adjustments and sacrifices. When you don't live where the care is needed, it can be especially difficult to feel that you are doing enough and what you are doing is important. Believe me, it usually is!

However close your family is, it can be difficult to decide who does what. Your brother may live nearer your relative, but may find it difficult to co-ordinate your relative's health care for example. The best way is to set up a family meeting. If you are unable to do this in person you may want to try Skype, a free piece of computer software that enables people who have it on their computer to see and speak to each other wherever they are in the world for free.

Think about how you can adapt your workload to provide respite for a primary carer or to co-ordinate a holiday. One long distance carer I know travelled to stay with their father, while the primary carer went on a family vacation.

Try to also think about what you are good at and how those skills might help in the current situation:

- Are you good at supervising and leading others?
- Are you good at communicating, finding information, keeping people up-to-date and keeping others motivated and positive, whether on the phone or the computer?
- Are you good at managing finances?
- Are you comfortable speaking with medical staff and knowing what to say to others?

When reflecting on your strengths you also need to think about:

- How often, financially and mentally can you afford to travel?
- Can you be calm and assertive when communicating from a distance?
- Are you emotionally prepared to reverse roles with your parent, taking care of them instead of your parent taking care of you?
- How will your decision to take on caring responsibilities, affect your work and home life?

Rona's Story

Rona lives in Canada while her mother lives in England. Rona visited her mother regularly and began to notice that she was finding it difficult to manage on her own and arranged for an agency to provide homecare and for meals to be delivered. A few months later her mother had a fall and was found on the floor. She was taken to hospital and it took some time for staff to track Rona down. The hospital discharge co-ordinator wanted her to come in person to discuss what her mother needed to return home, but Rona was unable to get away immediately. She remembered that when she last visited her mother, the hairdresser gave her a card with the contact details of a new service that had been set-up to provide support for people with elderly relatives. She contacted them and they provided someone to meet the hospital discharge co-ordinator. That person now visits her mother once a month and sends Rona emails with updates and recommendations.

Points to remember

If your elderly relative is eligible for public funding and the support you give is regular and substantial, you are entitled to a carer's assessment:

- Even if you live a long way from the person for whom you are caring.
- Even if your relative has not been assessed or is not receiving services.
- Whether you work full or part time.
- If you intend looking after your relative when they come out of hospital.

Did you know?

It has been calculated that the average woman spends as many (or more) years caring for one, or both of her parents, as she spent caring for her children.

12. FUNDING AND FINANCE MATTERS

In this chapter we will explore the different issues of funding care and support and the welfare benefits to which you and your relative may be entitled.

Long-term-care, however and wherever it is provided, is likely to be long term, substantial and extremely costly. For most people, funding the cost of long term care fees represents the second largest purchase of their lifetime after buying their home. Indeed, people are often in the same position of being first-time buyers when it comes to choosing 24-hour care and support.

I therefore find it surprising that, while many older people make wills and arrangements for their final wishes to be known, and some make sure that their funerals are already paid for, they have not really thought about whether they might need care and support and, if so, what they would want to happen and how it would be funded.

Throughout the years I worked for Social Services, I found that people were often surprised and alarmed to discover that they would have to pay towards some or all of their care and support as they confuse personal care at home or in a residential home with free NHS care.

Care and support services are means-tested and are not free to everyone. Most people have to pay something towards the cost of their care and some will have to pay for all of their care costs. It all depends on your relative's type and level of need and their financial circumstances.

Your relative may need to pay for all of their own care, or they may be entitled to local authority funding, NHS care (free) or have entitlements to welfare benefits to help pay for their care and support.

Some of the rules for the financial assessments are applied differently, based on whether your relative is considered to need care in their own home or in a residential home.

Where to start

The best place to start with determining what, if any, funding might be available is by referring your elderly relative to the Social (Adult) Services department at their local authority for an assessment of their needs. As part of this, Social Services will carry out a financial assessment to determine whether they will have to meet any, some, or all of the cost of their care.

Social Care Funding for residential care

At present, the law requires that people with savings of more than £23,250 (including the capital value of any property) will have to pay in full for the accommodation and personal care they receive in a care home. The system of charging for residential care is based on national guidance in England although, as you will see later, changes are planned in the coming years.

All Social Services have their own systems, allowances and procedures, although every person who is funded by Social Services is entitled to a personal allowance to spend as they choose. However, the Department of Health has stated that this should not be used to pay a top-up or for services that should be included by the home as part of the care service.

Different financial rules apply for couples and single people.

Care in a residential home can also be free for up to six weeks if it is arranged as part of 'intermediate care' after hospital treatment.

The first twelve weeks of residential care

During the first twelve weeks after Social Services has made an assessment, the value of your relative's property should be 'disregarded' in their calculations.

The purpose of this twelve-week disregard is to give your relative time to sell, let, or raise money on their property to fund care costs. A note of caution, though: if your relative claims Attendance Allowance and Social Services is making an increased contribution to their care fees, the allowance is withdrawn after the fourth week and reinstated at the end of the twelve week disregard period.

Choice and third party payments

Social Services have a maximum fee they are willing to pay for a care home, including a person's assessed contribution, based on their level of need and the type of home. If you, or your relative, want to go into a more expensive care home, this may be possible if you, or another third party, such as another relative, friend or charity pay the additional amount, for as long as your relative is in the home. Under the arrangement, the third party pays the difference between Social Services' usual maximum rate and the amount the care home charges (often called a 'top-up' or third party contribution).

If your relative has a shortfall between the amount the council is prepared to pay and the fees that the care home charge, you should not be pressured into paying a top-up fee. If you are thinking about paying a top-up for a relative, it is important to make sure beforehand that the local council is paying a reasonable rate to purchase the care required.

If you have agreed to pay a third party top-up towards care home fees, you will be asked either by the care home or the local council to enter into a third party contract with them. You should be made aware that the contract would be between yourself and the care home or the local council, not the older person in the home.

The council has a responsibility to check that you are able to keep up the payments for as long as the resident is in the care home, so they may ask for details of your finances. This is because it may be important for the council to ask what will happen to the third party contribution when the fees go up (usually on an annual basis) as any increase may not be shared with the council and your contribution, as the third party, will go up whenever the fees increase. You should also be aware that if you are unable to keep up the payments, your relative may have to move to a cheaper care home.

Sam's Story

When Sam's father was diagnosed with debilitative lung disease soon after his second stroke, it was agreed he should move into a care home. His father was on a low income, and he had minimal savings so Social Services had agreed to fund the placement. Sam looked around a number of homes but the one he liked best, which was only a few minutes walk from where he lived, so he could visit his father regularly, cost £150 a week more than Social Services were willing to pay. As his father had been in the Royal Navy, I suggested that he apply to one of the charities for ex-servicemen to see if they could help meet the shortfall. A contribution of £50 a week was agreed and Sam made up the difference himself. His father moved into the home and settled well, although, sadly, he passed away a few months later.

Deprivation of capital

Where the local authority believes that someone has transferred capital or ownership of a property, or made extravagant purchases in order to avoid paying care home fees, they may decide that 'deprivation of capital' has occurred. If the authority decides that this is the case, it will see your relative as still having the capital or property (notional capital) that they deprived themselves of and will include its full value in their financial assessment for care home fees.

There is no time limit on how far back the council can look at your relative's financial affairs to see if 'deprivation of capital' has occurred. Different factors need to be considered, such as, the reasons for the transfer/spending, the timing of the transfer, the intention (or perceived intention) behind the transfer, and whether or not it could be foreseen, at the time of the transaction, that it was likely that you would need to go into a care home in the future. Any decision by the council that 'deprivation of capital' has occurred should be 'reasonable' and should be based on the evidence available.

Self-funding for long term care

If your relative has assets above the capital threshold, currently £23,250, and can afford the full cost of care from their savings (assets) and income, they can make their own arrangements for admission to a care home of their choice and funding of the care they need.

Fees charged by care homes vary considerably so it is important to compare the fees of one home with other homes and check what services are included within the fees and what is charged for separately as extras. You need to compare apples with apples and not apples with pears.

As a 'self-funder' it is important that your relative seeks independent advice, support and guidance because research suggests that about 85% of those having to meet care cost themselves either get no advice or they receive advice that does not include information about all their care and funding options.

They can obtain basic advice about care options from organisations like Age UK, NHS Choices and the Alzheimer's Society. More in depth advice, personal support and practical help is available from care consultancies such as Relative Matters, Manage My Care and Breakell. You can find their details in the Helpful Resources section.

Specialist financial advice

Unfortunately people who fund their own care make major decisions with consequences for large amounts of personal expenditure, on the basis of little or no financial advice. Few people are even aware that specialist financial advice exists in this field.

It is important that your relative understands all the options for paying for long- term care as the cost will vary depending on its type, intensity, location and duration. For example, the cost of live-in care, or a place in a care home, will cost hundreds of pounds a week. Costs can vary across the country and different care homes will charge different amounts based on the level of care your relative needs, the quality of the accommodation and the area it is in.

Decisions that have such financial implications should be made with advice and only after considering the costs of alternatives. I therefore strongly recommend that you and your relative get financial advice from a qualified, accredited, specialist financial advisor as soon as the need for care arises and before making important life changing decisions.

Specialist care fees advice from a trusted financial advisor will help them understand their entitlement to payments and benefits and to plan and make well informed decisions about how best to meet care and support costs over the long term.

Specialist financial advice is available to guide people through their financial options as a self-funder. Advising older people about their financial circumstances and needs is a specialist area of independent financial advice requiring additional qualifications, competence and abilities. There may be a number of financial solutions to assist people to retain their savings/capital whilst paying for care.

The Society of Later Life Advisers (SOLLA) is a not-for-profit organisation which seeks to help older people choose a specialist independent financial advisor who has demonstrated their enhanced knowledge, skills and competence to deal with the particular issues of later life. SOLLA is a trusted organisation and, within the financial advice sector, later life accreditation is recognised as the benchmark for quality in advising older people. The SOLLA website allows you or your relative to search for accredited financial advisers specialising in long term care advice within their area.

Proposed changes for long term care funding

There are proposals to change the way care is paid for in the next few years. This includes:

- A £72,000 cap on lifetime residential care costs in 2016, calculated as the total cost of an individual's eligible needs for care, including the local authority's contribution.

- An increase in the assets threshold below which people will be entitled to state financial assistance with residential care will be increased from £23,520 to £118,000, including their property. It is estimated that only one in eight people will benefit from the charging cap and, moreover, the cap is only triggered once an individual has been assessed by the local authority as eligible for care (See Chapter 1).

- An option of joining a not-for-profit deferred payment scheme where the local authority pays the individual's residential care fees in return for a charge on their estate, without forcing the sale of their house during their lifetime. This will be available in 2015 and will probably work in the same way as drawdown mortgages, where care home fees are added on weekly rather than in a lump sum so as to accrue interest as slowly as possible.

- Care home residents having to pay £12,000 'hotel charge' for their daily living costs, if they are considered able to afford it.

However these proposals could be delayed or change if there is a change of political leadership at the next general election.

Community (social care) funding for non-residential care

Local authorities have discretion about charging for non-residential care (i.e. care at home) although they must abide by legal guidance.

How much your relative will have to pay towards their care will depend on their savings, benefits and income. For some services like Meals on Wheels there is a fixed cost.

If your local authority will pay for some or all of your relative's care, there are several ways it can do so. It could provide the care directly to them, either through its own staff or through an organisation that it has contracted with. However, your relative has the option to be more in control of the money and how it is spent on their care through Personal Budgets and direct payments.

Personal Budgets and Direct Payments

If your relative's local authority agrees to pay some or all of your relative's home care support, it should offer them the choice of receiving the money by way of a Personal Budget or direct payment, although some local authorities are lagging behind and have yet to make Personal Budgets available to its residents.

This option is not currently available if your relative is in residential care, but this is expected to change in the near future.

Other sources of funding for long term care

NHS Continuing Healthcare

NHS continuing healthcare, sometimes called fully funded NHS care, is free care outside of hospital that is arranged and funded by the NHS in a person's own home or a care home. It is only available for people who need on-going healthcare and meet strict eligibility criteria. To be eligible for NHS continuing healthcare, your relative must be assessed as having a 'primary health need', have a complex medical condition and substantial and on-going care needs.

If you think your relative may be eligible for NHS continuing healthcare, they will need to be assessed by a registered nurse.

From April 2014, anyone receiving NHS continuing healthcare will have a right to ask for a Personal Health Budget.

NHS Funded Nursing Care

NHS-funded nursing care is care provided by a registered nurse, paid for by the NHS, for people who live in a care home. The NHS make the payment directly to the care (nursing) home to fund care from registered nurses.

When visiting and considering different care homes with nursing, i.e. nursing homes, and discussing the fees charged by different homes, it is important to establish whether the care home fees being quoted are inclusive or exclusive of the NHS funded nursing care contribution in order to compare costs.

If you think your relative may be eligible for NHS funded nursing care they will need to be assessed by a registered nurse.

Intermediate care

Older people can usually be eligible for free intermediate care from the NHS and or Social Services. This is provided on a short-term basis, typically up to six weeks, and is intended to help people to recover from an injury or illness, and stay independent. Intermediate care is usually provided when people are being discharged from hospital, and may help someone to keep living in their own home rather than moving into a care home.

Attendance Allowance

Attendance Allowance is a non means-tested benefit payable if a person aged 65 and over needs help with personal care or requires supervision to avoid danger to them. It is paid at two rates: a Lower rate for people requiring care either during the day *or* night; and a Higher rate for people requiring care by day *and* night.

Many Attendance Allowance claims fail on first application but succeed on appeal, so don't give up!

A benefit claim pack is available from the Department of Work and Pensions (DWP) Benefits and Disability Advice Line on 0800 882 200; or you can apply on-line: www.dwp.gov.uk/eservice

Extra money if you're looking after your relative

Carer's allowances

If you care for your relative (day or night) for at least 35 hours a week, consider applying for Carer's Allowance. First, get a benefits check for you and the person you care for by phoning the Carers UK Advice Line on 0808 808 7777. Find out if it's in both your interests to claim, as getting Carer's Allowance could reduce the benefits of the relative you care for.

You are unlikely to get Carer's Allowance if your pension is over the benchmark, but you may be able to claim underlying entitlement to Carer's Allowance (known as Carer Premium). This can mean extra money each week for you when they are calculating how much Council Tax you need to pay and how much you may receive in Housing Benefit or Pension Credit. The claiming process is complicated so ring the advice line above for help.

Support from a charity

If you are unable to claim for anything, have you thought about asking a charity for help?

There are more than 170,000 charities in England and Wales alone with a total income of £52 billion. Many help people who worked in a certain industry, live in a certain area, or have a particular health problem.

My father did his National Service in the RAF, and the RAF Association (020 8286 6667) were a great support by providing subsidised respite care in one of their fabulous residential care homes. They also contributed towards the cost of putting a wet room in my parents' bungalow.

How to find a charity

- Visit turn2us.org.uk or call their free confidential helpline on 0808 802 2000.
- Call Charity Search 0117 982 4060, www.charitysearch.org.uk

- Ask at your library or Citizens Advice Bureau to look at *Charities Digest*.

Points to remember

- Long-term care, however or wherever it is provided, can be extremely costly, yet people rarely plan for it.
- If your relative is considering residential or nursing home care, it is in everyone's best interest to seek accredited financial advice to ensure that all options are explored and any remaining inheritance is protected.
- In order to afford their preferred home care service or care home and make their savings last as long as possible, it is important that your relative receives the benefits and payments for which they are eligible.

Did you know?

Up to 60% of people eligible for Attendance Allowance don't claim.

13. LEGAL MATTERS

In this chapter we will look at the legal framework for acting on a person's behalf, making wills and how to get legal advice.

Power of Attorney

Most of us know that making a will is important to record our wishes on death. However, we are less likely to consider the importance of recording our wishes should we become incapable during our lifetime.

It is commonly believed that family will be able to make decisions on our behalf if we are no longer able to make them ourselves, but this is not the case. Unless we legally nominate someone to act on our behalf, we will come under the control of the Court of Protection also known as the Office of the Public Guardian (OPG). Believe me you do not want to go down this route if you can avoid it. It is intrusive, frustrating and expensive.

I would, therefore, encourage you to advise your relative to arrange for a Lasting Power of Attorney (LPA) in case they should for any reason, become incapable of managing their affairs. In 2007 LPA replaced Enduring Power of Attorney (EPA), which allowed people to choose someone they trust, a son or daughter for example, to manage their financial affairs should they become unable to do this themselves sometime in the future.

There are two different types of LPA:

- A Property and Finance LPA allows an attorney, chosen by your relative, to look after all their finances. This might include paying their bills, collecting their income and benefits or selling their house if required.

- A Health and Welfare LPA allows people they choose to make important decisions about their welfare, but only if they become mentally or physically incapable of doing so themselves. If their health deteriorates then LPAs make the running of their life much easier for them.

An EPA made before 2007 is still valid but does not include decisions about medical treatment. This could present problems within a family that cannot agree on a course of treatment.

Nat's story

Nat had held an Enduring Power of Attorney (EPA) for his father since 2006. When his father had a stroke he was asked whether or not he wanted him to be resuscitated if his condition deteriorated. Nat believed that his father's quality of life was too poor to warrant intrusive treatment but his brother and sister believed that his life should be prolonged at all costs. As you can imagine the situation could have caused conflict within the family. Luckily Nat's father's condition improved and a decision did not have to be made.

If however, Nat's father had discussed his wish not to be resuscitated should he become seriously ill, while he was still well, he could have replaced the EPA with a Lasting Power of Attorney (LPA). The family would then have been able to make decisions like this, knowing they have carried out their father's wishes.

If you are appointed in your relative's LPA, make sure you are aware of their wishes about their finances and future medical care. This can feel difficult, so I would suggest you have the discussion with your relative when they are making arrangements for the LPA. If an EPA or LPA is already in place, plan the discussion when you have the time to talk the matter through thoroughly. Explain to your relative that you want to make sure that you carry out their wishes and in order to do so, need to discuss some difficult issues. It is a good idea to make notes so you have something you can refer back to at a later date. Make sure you keep them in a safe place, somewhere that you will remember, such as wherever you keep the LPA document.

It is important that your relative thinks about making a LPA while they still have mental capacity, as a LPA cannot be put in place once they lose mental capacity. They can choose anyone they trust so long as the person isn't bankrupt when they sign the papers.

You can download LPA forms from the website *www.guardianship.gov.uk*, or buy them from solicitors or high street stationers. Although you don't have to seek legal advice, a LPA is an important legal document, so you may want to seek advice from a solicitor who has experience of preparing them.

The Mental Capacity Act

The Mental Capacity Act 2005 provides a legal framework to protect people who may not be able to make decisions themselves. The Act sets out the decision making process for individuals who may not have capacity and enables people to plan ahead for such an eventuality.

The Act is underpinned by five key principles:

- A presumption of capacity – adults have the right to make their own decisions and, unless proven otherwise, must be assumed to have the capacity to do so.

- The right to be supported – everyone must be given appropriate help and support to make their own decisions, before anyone concludes that they cannot decide for themselves.

- Making the wrong decisions – individuals must retain the right to make what others may consider, eccentric or unwise decisions.

- Best interest – anything done for someone without capacity, must be done in their best interests.
- Least restrictive intervention – anything done for people without capacity, should be the least restrictive of their basic freedoms.

Advocacy

All Social Service departments are required to provide an independent mental capacity advocacy service to support people who have been assessed as having no capacity to make decisions about:

- Future long-term accommodation moves (such as from hospital to residential care).
- Serious medical treatment.
- Personal safety following an alert about suspected abuse.

An independent mental capacity advocate can be arranged through Social Services.

Deprivation of Liberty Safeguards

The Mental Capacity Act was extended in April 2009 to include extra legal safeguards. These "Deprivation of Liberty Safeguards" (DoLS) have been put in place for people who lack mental capacity and who live in care homes or hospitals. The safeguards or rules apply, irrespective of whether the care or treatment is being funded privately or by Social Services or the NHS.

DoLS have been put in place to ensure that people who lack capacity are treated and cared for in a way that means they are safe and free to do the things they want to do. If they are stopped from doing the things they want all the time, this is called being deprived of their liberty. Some examples of deprivation of liberty include:

- Staff in a care home or hospital having control over all the decisions in your relative's life.
- Not being able to leave the care home or hospital where they live.
- Family, carers or friends not being allowed to visit a relative.

My Story

Before going on holiday a few years ago, I arranged for my mother to stay in a care home to give my father a break while I was away. A couple of months after I returned she told me that she would never go there again. When I asked why, she said it was because staff had put cot sides up at night, which she hated as she was unable to get out of bed and use the toilet. Apparently, staff were concerned about the risk of her falling out of bed. Despite my mother telling them she would sign a disclaimer, they still refused to take away her cot sides at night. I made a formal complaint to the home and made sure Mum never went there again. Under the new safeguards, this would be considered as depriving my mother of her liberty and had it happened after April 2009, I would have reported the matter to the DoLS Team at Social Services. They would have undertaken a DoLS Best Interests Assessment and noted it as an adult safeguarding alert, as they would have been, by definition, highlighting a potential or actual infringement of my mother's human rights.

Making a will

If your relative does not already have a will I strongly advise you to encourage them to make one to ensure that their estate is distributed, as they would wish, after their death.

In cases where there is no will, or none that is valid, your relative would be said to have died 'intestate'. Beneficiaries are identified by the intestacy rules, which provide for a surviving spouse or children to receive a specific share of their estate. If there were no spouse or children, the siblings of your relative would inherit.

Age UK offers a guide to making a will on their website and also provide a wills advice service. Details of how to contact them are in Helpful Resources.

Whilst some people choose to make their own will, I believe it is better to have a solicitor who understands the different eventualities, which may arise. Some solicitors offer a "fixed fee" service for drawing up a will and if you shop around it needn't be expensive.

There are also certain times annually when solicitors offer promotional will-making campaigns as an incentive to us to make a will. For example an annual campaign organised by *Will Aid*, runs for the month of November, when participating solicitors can draw up a new will, oversee an existing will or add an amendment (codicil) to an existing will. In doing so the solicitors waive their fees and invite a donation to a *Will Aid* charity instead, ensuring funds are raised for exceptional work throughout the world. For further information and participating solicitors visit *www.willaid.org.uk*.

Your relative can make changes to the will subsequently, if their circumstances change or they simply change their mind. This is called a codicil and has to be witnessed in the same way as the original document.

Finally, make sure that you know where your relative's will is kept. They may have expressed their preferences for what happens to their body (burial or cremation) so you will need to check it on (or soon after) their death.

Obtaining legal advice

There are many reasons why your elderly relative might need legal advice including buying or selling their home, making a will or organizing a Lasting Power of Attorney. People who do not have a relative to help manage their affairs may also seek help from a solicitor to make arrangements to pay for their care.

Although you may be able to do some of these things for your relative, a solicitor may be able to spot a solution or avoid a problem that you haven't thought of. They are also more able to help you make your case in a more effective way as they have a better understanding of the law and how it works in practice.

It is also worth checking the conditions of your relative's bank account and house contents insurance to see if they include legal cover.

Points to remember

- It is important that your elderly relative arranges a Lasting Power of Attorney (LPA) to ensure someone they trust can make decisions for them, should they become incapable of managing their affairs in the future.
- Your relative needs to make a LPA while they still have mental capacity.
- Extra legal safeguards have been put in place to ensure that people who live in a care home or

hospital and lack capacity, are treated and cared for in a way that means they are safe and free to do the things they want to.

- A living will can be made to give specific instructions with regard to medical treatment should your relative fall ill. It can request life sustaining treatment or refusal of it.

- Your relative should make a will to ensure that their estate is distributed, as they would wish after their death.

Did you know?

In the UK, seven out of ten people die without making a will.

14. SAFEGUARDING MATTERS

In this chapter we will look at raising awareness about safeguarding adults, specifically older people, from abuse. This will include the people who might abuse an older person, why an older person might be abused, where an older person might be abused, the different types of abuse and how statutory services might help.

We all have the right to feel and be safe, regardless of our age or circumstances, so you may be surprised to know that reported incidents of abuse towards older people are increasing, in addition to many that are not reported. Even more surprisingly, a UK study undertaken in 2007 demonstrated that those closest to older people are often the ones most likely to commit abuse. It is therefore important that we are vigilant to ensure our relatives, their property and belongings are safe and they are treated with the dignity and respect they have a right to and deserve.

Abuse can occur anywhere, for example in a person's own home, in a care or nursing home, day centre, sheltered accommodation or a hospital. The perpetrators of abuse can be a relative, friend or neighbour, someone who provides support, such as a care worker, or a stranger.

All Social Services departments must have clear procedures about how they will safeguard vulnerable adults, which should show how organisations should work together, and communicate effectively. Social Services have Safeguarding Teams with responsibility for investigating allegations of abuse, which are called "safeguarding alerts".

The charity, *Action on Elder Abuse*, defines abuse as: "A single or repeated act or lack of appropriate action, occurring within any relationship where there is an expectation of trust, which causes harm or distress to another person".

Abuse is a complex issue and often involves more than one type of abuse. For example financial abuse may also involve emotional abuse if someone is being threatened as well as complying with inappropriate demands for money.

An understanding of situations that may create a risk of abuse is necessary so that you can identify the signs before they escalate. However you need to balance this in order that your relative's choices are respected, if they have the capacity to make them.

The opinions and choices of your relative should guide the action to be taken where abuse is involved.

You also need to consider what happens after an abuse situation. This can be difficult if the person, who causes the abuse, is very close to your relative and may have an on-going relationship with them.

Let's look at the different categories of abuse you are likely to come across in relation to older people in a bit more detail so you know what you are looking for.

Physical abuse

Physical abuse is where someone intentionally inflicts injury, pain or bodily harm on another person. It can also result in psychological problems and feelings of fear.

Examples of behaviour include: hitting, pushing, slapping, scalding, shaking, pushing, kicking, pinching, hair pulling, the inappropriate application of techniques or treatments, involuntary isolation or confinement and misuse of medication. Inadvertent physical abuse may also arise from poor practice such as poor manual handling techniques.

Possible signs of physical abuse are:

- Cuts
- Scratches
- Bite marks
- Puncture wounds
- Finger marks
- Burns and scalds
- Weal marks
- Fractures and sprains
- Any injury that has not been properly cared for such as undressed pressure sores
- Poor skin condition
- Bruises (especially if there is a lot of bruising of different ages illustrated by varying levels of discolouration)
- Loss of weight, loss of hair and change of appetite
- Unexplained behaviour
- Changes in sleep pattern
- Unexplained paranoia
- Fearfulness
- Anxiety

Roy's Story

Roy has dementia and lives with his daughter, Joan, and son-in-law, Pete. Roy frequently becomes anxious and seeks reassurance from Joan, often repeating his questions over and over again because of his poor short-term memory. Joan has been worried recently about Pete's business, which has been losing money because of the recession. She has taken on a part-time job in the evenings when Pete is home to look after Roy and she has been feeling very tired as her father's demands on her have been increasing. Joan has found herself getting increasingly frustrated with her father and has shaken him on occasions, more than once leaving finger marks on his arms. As a result Roy has lost his appetite and has become quiet and withdrawn.

Financial abuse

Financial abuse can been described as: "the unauthorised and improper use of funds, property or any resources belonging to an individual" or "the illegal or unauthorised use of a person's money, property or other valuables". Crimes associated with financial abuse include theft, forgery and undue influence.

Those who financially abuse may be people who hold a position of power or authority or have the confidence of the vulnerable person. It could involve pressure being put on an elderly person to lend or give money to friends, relatives or the professionals working with them. Pressure could be exerted to change their will or sign over property; a family member could take charge of an individual's pension and not give them all the money, or cash a cheque without permission. An elderly person could be charged an excessive amount for a service such as decorating or mending a roof.

Possible signs of financial abuse are:
- Unusual activity in bank accounts
- Unexplained loss of money
- Deterioration in standard of living, for example not being able to pay for things they could previously afford
- Person unable to access their own money to check their own account
- Sudden change or creation of a will to benefit someone significantly
- Inappropriate granting and/or use of a Power of Attorney

- Cheques being cashed without the person's consent
- Missing personal belongings such as jewellery

Examples of financially abusive behaviour include: misappropriating money, valuables or property, forcing changes to a will, preventing access to money, property, possessions or inheritance and stealing.

Celia's Story

Celia has diabetes and had a stroke a year ago; since then she has been confused. An agency provides care workers to visit three times a day to provide personal care and ensure she eats regularly. Celia pays for this care herself out of her savings. Her grandson Lorrie, visits regularly, pays her bills and manages Celia's money for her. Lorrie decides to reduce the number of visits from three times a day to once a day and rings the agency to let them know. The agency calls the Safeguarding Team at Social Services. They report that Celia needs three visits to ensure that she eats regularly to maintain her sugar levels and are concerned that something is wrong.

Neglect

Neglect is a form of abuse whereby people responsible for providing care for someone who is unable to look after themselves, fail to meet their needs. Neglect can be intentional or can occur as a result of not understanding what the person's needs are. Under the Mental Capacity Act 2005, wilful neglect and ill treatment become a criminal offence.

Self-neglect on the part of the person does not usually lead to a safeguarding alert, unless the situation involves a significant act of omission by someone with responsibility for the person's care. A person who is unable to look after themself is put at risk by being left unattended.

Neglect occurs when there is failure to provide food, shelter, clothing, heating, medical care, hygiene or personal care, and the inappropriate use of medication. Examples could include not giving someone proper assistance with eating and drinking, or failure to provide a warm, safe and comfortable environment, or failing to provide adequate personal care, ignoring someone's health needs – including a failure to give medication as prescribed by the person's GP. Repeated calls for assistance may be ignored or someone's care plan may not be read or followed.

Possible signs of neglect are:

- Urine smell in a person's environment
- Pressure sores
- Depression
- Lack of stimulation or prolonged isolation
- Person has unkempt appearance or is dressed inappropriately
- Signs of malnourishment or dehydration
- Person has untreated medical condition
- Not being helped to the toilet when assistance is requested.
- Home has insufficient or no heating
- Under or over medication.

Paula's Story

Rose has Alzheimer's and lives in a specialist care home for people with dementia. Her only relative, Paula, is unable to visit very often as she lives more than a hundred miles away and works long hours. When Paula visits her aunt she is concerned to find that Rose does not have her own dress on and it is too big for her. Her hair had been cut badly and has not been styled and her lower dentures are missing. Paula is aware of a strong smell of urine in the home and observed that her aunt was wearing an incontinence pad that needed changing. The most worrying thing for Paula was that her aunt appeared depressed and withdrawn.

Emotional/psychological abuse

Emotional or psychological abuse involves the use of threats, bullying, humiliation, swearing or any form of mental cruelty that results in mental or physical distress. It includes the denial of basic human and civil rights, such as choice, self-expression, privacy and dignity.

Emotional or psychological abuse could consist of not respecting a person's right to privacy and dignity; for example leaving the toilet door open when assisting someone to use the toilet in a communal setting or failing to knock on their door before going in. It could involve humiliation, for example making a person feel ashamed of their behaviour, or the way they act, through words or actions that make the person feel unimportant, unworthy, unwanted or ignored. A person's wishes could be denied, for example their choice of food or clothing. This could be particularly significant if the choice has a particular religious or cultural meaning to the person.

Examples of emotionally abusive behaviour include: treating a person in an inappropriate way for their age and/or cultural background, blaming, swearing, intimidation, insulting, harassing, deprivation of contact, cold-shouldering.

Possible signs of emotional or psychological abuse:
- Anger or aggression
- Untypical changes in mood and behaviour
- Loss of appetite
- Helplessness or passivity
- Changes in sleep pattern
- Confusion or disorientation
- Fear and anxiety

You should be aware that there might be other reasons for these signs in any given situation.

Maud's Story

When her husband died, Maud went to live with her son and daughter-in-law as she had severe arthritis and needed help with daily living tasks. A care worker from a local agency came twice a day to help Maud with her personal care and to get dressed and undressed.

There is tension in the house and Maud's daughter-in-law has become resentful of the amount of time Maud is taking. She has started shouting at Maud to "hurry up", calling her a "lazy cow" and taking over doing things for her. Maud now feels anxious and depressed and has become withdrawn. She has also lost most of her remaining independence.

Institutional abuse

Institutional abuse arises from repeated instances of poor care of individuals or groups of individuals. It occurs when there is poor professional practice as a result of routines, systems and policies within a care setting, which override the needs of the people they are there to support.

It can occur in any setting where one person or more receive a service on a daily or residential basis, for example in a person's own home, a day centre, care home or hospital ward. The service may not meet the necessary professional standards or there is a training need for a more personalised approach.

Examples of behaviour include: inflexible routines set around the needs of staff rather than people using the service, for example requiring everyone to eat together at specific times, limiting bathing to times that suit staff rather than the individual and no doors on toilets. These situations can arise through lax, uninformed or punitive management regimes. The behaviour is cultural and not specific to a particular member of staff.

Possible signs of institutional abuse are:

- Set times for refreshments with no opportunity to make alternative arrangements outside these hours
- Inappropriate approaches to continence issues such as toileting at prescribed times as opposed to when a person wishes to use the toilet
- No evidence of care plans that focus on an individual's specific needs
- Staff not following care plans
- Lack of privacy, such as leaving the door open when someone is taken to the toilet

- Dehumanising language that does not treat a person with dignity and respect
- Abuse of medication
- Locking people in rooms
- Failure to promote or support an individual's religious or cultural needs
- No access to personal allowance or personal possessions
- Failure to knock on a person's bedroom or bathroom door before entering
- A couple being prevented from living together
- Inflexible visiting times

Maisey's Story

Maisey is confined to a wheelchair and lives in a care home. She does not like wearing pads and, to avoid having an accident, needs to be taken to the toilet as soon as she feels the need to go. While this is made clear in Maisey's care plan, staff regularly ignore her requests to use the toilet until it is too late. When she complains about this to staff she is told it's because she always asks when they are busy doing other things and, while they respect her choice not to wear pads, if she did so accidents could be avoided.

Discriminatory abuse

Discriminatory abuse is where a person is abused or treated less favourably because of their race, gender, ethnicity or culture, disability, sexual orientation, age or political views. It could involve withholding services or treatment from an elderly person, a presumption of a lack of capacity without proper justification, expecting a person to eat food that is unacceptable to their faith or failing to take account of the spiritual welfare of a person when providing palliative care.

Examples of discriminatory behaviour include; unequal treatment, verbal abuse, inappropriate use of language, slurs, harassment or deliberate exclusion.

Denise's Story

Denise is profoundly deaf and devoutly religious. Before being admitted to hospital for planned surgery, her family gave staff information about her religious practice, which included the fact that she does not eat a certain type of meat. Following admission, Denise is distressed when she is given that meat and when she tries to indicate this to staff they ignore her.

All of these abuse categories have the potential to involve illegal activity. Social Services work jointly with other agencies, such as the Police, Crown Prosecution Service, Care Quality Commission, voluntary organisations and the NHS. Where abuse involves criminal activity Social Services will refer the matter to the police, who will expect to lead the investigation.

What to do if you suspect that your relative is being abused

If you become suspicious that your relative is being abused because you have observed changes in their behaviour or living patterns it is important that you do not ignore it.

You need to talk to them about what you suspect in a calm and sensitive way and help them realise that there are people who can help them. You need to be honest with them and ask what they would like to do about it. Your relative might not want to take any action at first and it may take a while before they agree to you taking the matter forward on their behalf. If your relative lacks mental capacity to make the decision, you can make it for them by acting in their best interest.

When you refer an abuse situation to Social Services it is known as an "Adult Safeguarding Alert". Social Services will arrange to have the matter investigated according to the level of risk to your relative and should keep you both informed about progress.

The contact details for your relative's Social Services department, which is part of their local council, will be listed in the telephone directory under the name of their council.

If your relative has been subjected to abuse and feels they require independent support to help them through the process and to ensure their wishes are heard, you can contact a local voluntary service such as *Age UK* or the *Alzheimer's Society* who may provide, or put you in touch, with an independent advocacy service.

Points to remember

- Your relative has a right to be kept safe and treated with dignity and respect.
- It is important to be aware of the different types of abuse and what to look out for.

- If you suspect that your relative has been abused it is important that you talk to them about it. If they choose to take the matter forward you need to report the matter to the Safeguarding Team at Social Services.

- If your relative lacks mental capacity to make the decision about whether to report suspected abuse to Social Services, you can make it for them by acting in their best interest.

- Social Services have Safeguarding Teams with responsibility for investigating allegations of abuse called "safeguarding alerts".

Did you know?

A UK study found that, in the previous year, 342,400 people aged over sixty-six years, living in private households, reported mistreatment by a family member, close friend, care worker or neighbour.

15. FAMILY AND EMOTIONAL MATTERS

In this chapter we will catch up with my parents' journey, explore what family is, why we need our family and consider the emotional perspective of caring for our elderly relatives.

My mother is waiting to move into her new care home and looking forward to it. I was with her when the new manager carried out her assessment and was impressed when she referred to the home being "for people with memory problems" when Mum asked if it was a "mental home". I was also reassured by the time she spent recording the things that are important to and for Mum and the myriad small things that make her the wonderful, unique person she is. The room my mother is moving into is being decorated and a new carpet put down so it will be nice and fresh for her. My brother and sister are busy putting together Mum's life story in pictures in order that she can reflect on happy memories rather than depressing thoughts. The staff will also be able to get to know her as an interesting person rather than someone with dementia.

My father is now very frail, increasingly forgetful and unable to process and retain information. He has to deal with chronic health problems and the loss of his sight as well as the emotional impact of being separated from his wife of sixty-four years. Despite his many challenges, Dad remains positive, and counts himself lucky to have been able to travel so much and enjoy a happy marriage. I never tire of listening to the many interesting stories about his life and am currently on a mission to get the war medals, of which he is so proud, remounted for him.

I am finding caring for my parents in separate places more demanding than before and emotionally draining. Mum is overtly needy, while Dad rarely asks for anything, is fiercely proud and independent and doesn't want to trouble anyone. However, he is every bit as needy as my mother and I regularly have to play detective, use my observation and listening skills, and craft careful questions to ensure his needs are met.

Reflecting on my situation, and although I regard caring for my parents a privilege, when I am in the middle of the situation life sometimes feels very hard. There has also been occasional tension between wanting to do my best for my parents and wanting to live my own life. Taking responsibility for the welfare of someone else and treating them with respect and dignity has a huge impact on our life. However, there are good times too and the time I spend caring for my parents will leave many fond memories by which to remember them.

Now, as my parents are elderly, fragile and unable to be as independent as they once were, it is also very sad for me. My heart feels like breaking when I realise that it is only a matter of time before I will no longer have them in my life, physically anyway. However, I know there are many people in the same boat as my brother, sister and me. Being part of a loving family that support each other during difficult times is something that I value highly and the thing that enables me to keep going with a degree of sanity.

What is family?

The word "family" can mean different things to different people and families come in different shapes and sizes. Your family might be the family you were born into or the family you have created with your partner. You might include just your partner or families that one or both of you bring from previous relationships.

Families may be based on different kinds of adult relationships but the one thing they have in common is that they provide a sense of belonging. They give identity and provide security and support. The family is where vulnerable family members should be able to go for safety and support.

However we think about family, most share common values. Values are something we don't often think or talk about and yet they are always there, shaping the way we behave towards one another. Our values are what we draw on to cope with the ups and downs of family life and will play a big part in how we care for older family members.

What values do you hold about family? To identify what values you hold, grab a piece of paper and jot down as many answers as you can to the following questions.

- What is most important to me about family?
- Are there things your family believed in the past that you would like to go back to?
- Or are they values held by previous generations that no longer fit your life?

When you start thinking along these lines it's likely that you will come up with a set of fairly common principles. For instance, most of us would say we trust one another, support one another, care for each other when the going gets tough and make sure that everyone in the family is safe.

In addition to shared values it is also important to consider culture. England is now a cosmopolitan country and there are many different cultures with beliefs and values that are very different to our own. I was unexpectedly exposed to a different culture and how families behave when one of them becomes ill.

While on a holiday to Greece, I was taken ill and admitted to hospital for a couple of weeks. This was an interesting experience and I watched fascinated while family members took it in turns to carry out basic nursing tasks for their loved ones throughout the day and night, leaving nurses to focus exclusively on medical treatments.

Whenever possible I would try and communicate with relatives, in order to gain insight to their culture and the motivation behind what were often prolonged and intensive visits over several days. I watched with interest as older women waddled in with stooped backs and weary walks, probably the result of lifting and caring for their elderly relatives without a hoist or care workers to help them. I was told that staying with their loved one while they were in hospital was a way to show their relative how much they loved them. Despite it robbing them of time that was often needed elsewhere, they would feel they were letting the person down if they did not make sure someone was looking after them for the whole time they were in hospital.

We each have a unique purpose within our family. My siblings and I play different roles in caring for our parents and each of us handles the situation differently. Indeed there are as many different ways of dealing with the care of an ageing parent as there are people.

My brother, who is eight years younger than me, has a particularly close relationship with our mother, which began when he was born with a deformed foot. Mum would not accept that he would remain in callipers for the rest of his life and manipulated his foot three times a day for two years. This made him scream and be would plead with her to not to do it. However, to the astonishment of the doctors, she persevered and my brother has never worn a calliper!

He apparently invented the word "procrastination" and avoids confrontation like the plague. He has a heart of gold, takes our father to have lunch with Mum every week and will take either parent anywhere they need or want to go if he is not working; that includes taking them on holiday, which is jolly hard work.

My younger sister, who is also my best friend, lives sixty miles away and leads a busy life working and looking after her family. She lacks driving confidence and relies on my brother-in-law for driving to visit Mum and Dad. My sister is a great listener and provides a wise and receptive sounding board when I need to let off steam or gain a different perspective on things.

I am the eldest and have worked in the caring services for many years. As a result I am the organiser, consultant, negotiator, coordinator, mediator, financial assistant, employer and service coordinator for our parent's care. However, caring for our parents is very much a team effort and I rely on my brother and sister to support my efforts.

Caring isn't easy. However much care we give our elderly loved ones, decline in strength and health is usually painful and it can be very discouraging to know this is happening despite our best efforts. Like many areas of life, there are no magic formulas or training manuals and we just have to strive to do our best. Also remember, it is quite normal to feel lonely, misunderstood, unappreciated and angry about what is happening to the people we love.

Sometimes it becomes necessary to make unpopular decisions about "what is best" for people we love dearly. This can make us feel as if we are betraying them or letting them down in some way. This was certainly the case when the decision was made that my mother needed to go into a care home. Although we considered every possible alternative option and I knew there was no other way Mum could be looked after because of her obsessive dependence on my father, I felt so guilty at being unable to come up with a solution that would have enabled them to stay together. Guilt is an emotion commonly associated with caring for an elderly relative and it can sometimes cause us to delay making a decision, until suddenly it reaches a crisis.

The decision on whether to move into a care home is usually taken in circumstances nobody would choose and we have to ask ourselves: "Was there really an alternative?" There are many reasons, which could lead up to the event, and there are all kinds of complexities and difficult relationships within families. As relatives we have to make decisions that balance competing obligations and pressures, which are capable of being sustained in the long term.

During the time I was responsible for managing care homes for older people, I was acutely aware that when a parent, partner or other relative moves into a care home, guilt is a commonly felt emotion. For some of us this feeling is inevitable, but acknowledging it and thinking through why we feel this way can help us accept it.

Genuine guilt is a useful feeling when it results from a true fault. However the feelings of guilt we can often be plagued with are coming from our perception of what someone else might think about what we are doing, which is not helpful.

Lynn and Stuart's Story

Lynn's mother Doris, was adamant that she did not want to leave her home and move into a care home. As Doris became more confused she needed a care worker to go in twice a day. Every time care workers or a visiting family member left Doris, she cried because she felt lonely. On reflection, Lynn wished she had ignored her mothers' pleas to remain at home and coaxed her to move into a care home.

When Lynn's father Jack had a stroke he needed 24-hour care in a nursing home. Every time she visited, Jack asked if she had come to take him home.

Lynn felt heartbroken every time she left him there. If she could have had Jack home with her she would.

After Doris and Jack passed away Lynn became overcome with guilt when she thought about how she could have done things differently for her parents.

It can be a kind of bereavement when a loved one has to move into a care home, especially if you have been involved with caring for them. Handing over responsibility, even if the move is an acknowledgement that the responsibility is too great (as was the case with my father) can be a very difficult process.

When we try to find the best solution in challenging circumstances it can trigger a sense of despair, helplessness or even panic. There may be pressure from others such as the hospital discharge co-ordinator, asking us to make arrangements quickly. This pressure can mean that with the benefit of hindsight, you may feel that you have made a decision that was second best or inadequate in some way. However always remember that while not to be undertaken lightly, you can always move your relative to another care home or back home if that is possible and appropriate.

The changes that have to be made as a result of decisions we make can be hard for us as well as our relative. In the case of our parents, we may also feel their role has changed and they are now no longer there for us as they were in the past. This change in roles can be stressful as it causes uncertainty.

While it is important to acknowledge our thoughts and feelings we need to remind ourselves that our relative has gone through a much bigger ordeal. Even if they have difficulty expressing themselves, they are probably experiencing their own bereavement for loss of family and friends, and for some, their own home and independence.

When it comes to being responsible for someone else's care, especially someone we love, anything less than perfect may feel unacceptable and inexcusable. This often happens when we are caring for a loved one. Our life revolves around caring for that person and it can feel like an overwhelming task.

Caring for and about an elderly family member who is unable to look after themself can be very stressful. Stress has nothing to do with how much we love our family member. We can love someone and still be aware of frazzled nerves. The key to staying as stress-free as possible is to recognise when it is trying to creep up on us.

Here are some signs to watch out for:

- Becoming short tempered
- Feeling tired all the time
- Increased incidence of illness
- Weight gain or loss
- Headaches
- Anxiety or depression.

When showing signs of stress it is important that you get the help you need. Stress is a part of our everyday life, but the level of stress depends on our coping mechanisms. If anyone ever needed good coping mechanisms, it's a carer!

Here are some ways to give yourself a break to put the pieces back together:

- Consult and ask other family members to share responsibility.
- Delegate. Find ways to outsource certain tasks to lighten your load. Consider using *Meals-on-Wheels* (they are much better than they used to be), day-care to give you a break during the day or how about paying someone to do your housework or ironing to free up some of your time?

- Co-ordinate with a family member or friend to care for your loved one while you head out for a weekend break to rest and recharge your batteries.

- Stay physically active. Stress can weaken our immune system. When we stay active, we build it back up and increase endorphin production, which gives us a sense of positive well-being.

- Give yourself a treat like a massage or treatment.

- Build regular "me time" into your daily routine.

- Take up meditation or yoga.

- Join a support group. Just being with others who understand what you are going through can help you breathe a sigh of relief. They may be able to make suggestions you hadn't thought of to decrease stress. Most carers' organisations offer group meetings or support groups.

Points to remember

- Family gives us a sense of identity and, for most of us, provides security and support.

- We need to acknowledge guilt and think through why we are feeling guilty, in order to accept it.

- Caring for a loved one can be stressful so it is important we put strategies in place to look after ourselves.

Did you know?

Fifty-two percent of carers have been treated for stress because of their caring role.

16. DEMENTIA MATTERS

In this chapter we will revisit my parents' story and consider dementia and how it has impacted on my mother's life as well as the rest of our family.

I have learned to accept my mother's confused and distorted view of reality and come to accept that there is little point in increasing her anxiety and my own frustration by trying to change her perception. However, it is still not easy to hear her agonising about my father having gone off without telling her where he has gone. Nor that he cannot love her anymore because he is living in their home, while she is having to live "in this place". Visits and phone conversations with Mum have become a strain for my father who struggles to understand how to respond to her and forgets his doctor's advice to humour or distract Mum rather than try to make her understand.

After a particularly difficult weekend, I contacted her psychiatrist. I knew Mum had dementia because she had been diagnosed nearly thirty years ago at a London hospital. I was also aware that there are many forms of dementia and wanted to know which type Mum had in order to understand her behaviour better and how best to manage it.

What he said shook me to the core. He told me that Mum has Alzheimer's. It had never crossed my mind that the dementia Mum was diagnosed with all those years ago, could have developed into Alzheimer's.

Dementia is usually caused by illness or mini-strokes that have damaged a person's brain cells and the term "dementia" is used to describe the symptoms that occur when the brain is affected by specific diseases and conditions (of which depression is one). According to the *Alzheimer's Society*, there are more than a hundred different types of dementia, all of which are progressive. This means that the structure and chemistry of the brain becomes increasingly damaged over time.

I have managed specialist care homes for older people suffering from dementia and the residents were at a more advanced stage of the disease than my mother. I was also responsible for a specialist day centre and home care service for people who were at the mid-stage of their dementia journey. Having worked with people who have Alzheimer's, I would say that Mum's behaviour is definitely not typical, although I am aware that it affects people differently.

There are drugs available that appear to alleviate some of the symptoms in the early stages of Alzheimer's for some people. Other treatments are not automatically available in all parts of the country due to Primary Care Trusts differing interpretation of decisions made by the National Institute of Clinical Excellence (NICE). This results in a "post code lottery" for some medication.

Here are some tips that I found helpful when looking after people living with dementia

- Learn from the person themselves – they are the experts on their disability.
- Plan more active days for your relative. Consider finding someone to do activities with them or use a specialist day care service.
- Keep to a set routine as much as possible. Try to replicate the routine your relative maintained during the majority of their life.
- Encourage a rest period after lunch to reduce afternoon fatigue.
- If your loved one is experiencing a delusion or hallucination, don't try to convince them that

they're wrong. Just go along with it and reassure them that they are safe and loved.

- Don't interrupt them. Agree/acknowledge everything they say.
- Don't ask questions. It confuses them.
- Make afternoon and evening hours less hectic. Schedule appointments, trips and activities, such as baths or showers, early in the day.
- Avoid asking what the problem is. They will not be able to tell you.
- Reduce the level of noise from radios, televisions or stereos.
- Try playing calming music and do something soothing and relaxing with your relative, such as giving them a hand massage.
- Limit the number of choices you give your elderly relative. Too much choice can create stress for them.

I have noticed that Mum frequently becomes agitated and confused and suffers from delusions during the evening more than during the day. This pattern of becoming agitated and confused is called Sundowners Syndrome, also known as Sundowning, which refers to a symptom often associated with the early stages of dementia, including Alzheimer's. Sufferers experience periods of extreme agitation during the late afternoon or early evening. Its exact cause is unknown. Some think it is a malfunction of the internal biological clock, while more recent research has raised the possibility of more organic causes such as drug interaction or stress associated with a dementia sufferer's condition. You can be reassured, however; Sundowning is a transient phase of the dementia process and will pass.

I first became aware of the behaviour associated with Sundowning when Mum rang me one evening in an agitated state and told me that my father had gone out again and not told her where he was going. This was something that he would never have done. I tried to reassure her that Dad was at home but she would have none of it claiming he was probably out with "that man". When I asked who she meant, she said "John, of course". John is my father's Personal Assistant (carer). Mum appeared to hear nothing I said so I reassured her that she was safe and told her that I loved her. These kind of calls from Mum during the evening became common and happened four or five times a week.

When I returned from my holiday, elongated by two weeks because I was taken ill and admitted to hospital, Mum appeared more depressed, anxious and confused than she had before I left. After a few weeks I went to look at some specialist care homes for people with dementia and found one that I thought would suit Mum. There were more staff on duty than at her current home and the staff receive regular training to help them understand dementia and how to manage what, at times, can be very difficult behaviour. Mum loves animals and the home was pet friendly, having two cats, a number of birds and three tortoises. Most importantly, I liked the attitude and approach of the manager, who respected her residents as individuals and treated them with dignity and respect. I also liked the way staff interacted with the residents. There was a real "buzz" in the home and I observed plenty of kindness and laughter.

I did some research on the Care Quality Commission (CQC's) website and spoke to some of my social work contacts. I was pleased to find that the home reportedly provides high standards of care and had an excellent reputation. My search was over. I had found the right home for Mum for a second time.

My brother wasn't quite ready to accept that Mum needed more specialised care although, following reflection and further discussion, came to accept it. My father and sister shared my views that

Mum needed to be cared for by people who understand her mental health issues.

In order for Social Services to agree the funding, I asked Mum's psychiatrist to confirm his diagnosis of dementia in writing to Social Services, with a recommendation that a specialist home would be better able to meet her needs. As soon as her social worker received this we were ready to take the next step, which was for the new home's manager to assess Mum to make sure the home could meet her needs. We then gave notice to the home she was in, which although usually four weeks, was mutually agreed at three weeks as it brought us neatly to the end of the month.

Despite Mum's agitation during the evening, we sometimes wonder if we made the right decision to move her to a specialist care home. One day she appears almost normal, intelligent, articulate and reasonable; on others, she is belligerent, angry, confused and hurt at being "abandoned" by my father. Whichever state she is in, her faithful companions, anxiety and depression, remain with her and sometimes she is unhappy, which is distressing. I have to repeatedly remind myself that it is not my job to make Mum happy, like each and every one of us, she has to take responsibility for that herself.

My father, siblings and I experienced a range of emotions about my mother's diagnosis. We are all trying to let go of the wife and mother we used to know and love and try and get to know the person she has and will become. It is not easy for any of us, especially my father.

One day Mum rang me out of the blue and said: "Tell me yes or no. Have I got Alzheimer's?" I was taken aback and had to think on my feet. I have always promised my parents I would tell them the truth so I told her as sensitively as I could what the psychiatrist had told me when I asked him what kind of dementia she had. I suggested that she might want to discuss it with him the next time he came to see her. She appeared to take the news well and told me she appreciated my honesty and has never mentioned it again.

We all found the situation stressful. It is easy to forget our own needs when caring for someone with dementia and we have to be mindful not to forget to safeguard our own health and well-being so we can continue to care for the people we love. It can be hard to watch someone we care about slip into being a person we no longer recognise and it can be distressing. We need to remember that we don't have to cope with this on our own. There are organisations out there that offer support groups and provide information and on-line forums to relatives of people with dementia, in particular the *Alzheimer's Society*. You can find their details in Helpful Resources.

I am acutely aware that we will soon have to watch the mother we love slip away as she changes, possibly quite dramatically, into someone we no longer know. We will then begin a period of bereavement when we will have to come to terms with the knowledge that we have "lost" the mother we knew and loved and someone else has replaced her. I have heard about this from many relatives over the years and will now experience it for myself.

I found the following advice helpful and hope if your elderly relative has dementia, you do too.

"You will need to travel light, and learn how to be flexible, to find new routes to familiar places, to throw away all of the old maps, all of the old guides. You are on a trip that will demand all of your patience, your stamina and your love."

Tom and Karen Brenner

Alzheimer's Reading Room

Points to remember

- There are over a hundred kinds of dementia, the most common of which is Alzheimer's.
- Dementia affects everyone differently.
- There are drugs available for some people in the early stages but the practice of prescribing them varies across the country.
- If a relative has dementia, there is help available by way of information, support groups and respite services.

Did you know?

Dementia is one of the main causes of disability in later life, ahead of some cancers, cardiovascular disease and stroke.

17. END OF LIFE MATTERS

In this chapter we will focus on: end of life planning; living wills, advance directives and advance statements; finding your relatives' important documents; end of life care; practical arrangements after a death; loss and bereavement.

End of life planning

Many of us worry about the time when our loved one's life will come to an end and how we can support them in the best way possible to die with dignity, ideally in a place of their choosing. To achieve this means helping our relatives to look ahead at possible future options for their healthcare, particularly at the end of their life. This means having a conversation with them to find out what their preferences are because In order to do any of these things, or just to support our elderly relative at the end of their life, we need to know what their wishes are.

Planning for end of life needs to begin before your relative's health becomes too poor and when they are still able to make their own decisions. Of course, this is not always possible if they have been diagnosed with a serious illness such as advanced cancer, if they have been taken ill or are unable to recover following surgery.

Living wills, advance directives and advance statements

When your relative becomes ill, they can usually discuss treatment options with their doctor and jointly reach a decision about their future care. However, if they had a car accident, a stroke, or developed dementia they may be unable to communicate their wishes. In this situation, doctors have a legal and ethical obligation to act in their perception of the person's best interests unless an advance directive to refuse treatment has been made. Medical professionals are bound to follow it, providing the decision is valid and relevant in the circumstances, whether or not they think it is in the person's best interests.

Advance directives and advance statements are formal names for the two types of "Living Will", which doesn't have a legal meaning. It is a statement expressing a person's views on how they would or would not like to be treated if they are unable to make a decision about their treatment themself sometime in the future.

An advance directive is a decision to refuse treatment and an advance statement is any other decision about how an individual would like to be treated.

An advance directive or statement may be in any of the following forms:

- A signed document or card. (If it is an advance refusal of treatment it must be witnessed).
- A witnessed oral statement.
- A discussion note recorded in their medical file, at your relative's request.

It may give specific instructions with regard to medical treatment should your relative fall ill and can request life sustaining treatment or refusal of it. In order to be legally binding a living will must meet the following requirements regarding the person at the time it is signed:

- Has the mental capacity to make the medical decisions contained in the living will.

- Understands the consequences of these decisions.
- Makes clear their wishes regarding future treatment (and the document covers the medical circumstances which later arise).
- Makes the decision(s) voluntarily and not under somebody else's influence.

Here are some definitions that are important for you and your relative to know about in relation to a Living Will.

Life prolonging treatments

These include cardio pulmonary resuscitation (heart and lung), artificial feeding and hydration, breathing by a machine, and intravenous medicine administered by a drip or injection.

Basic Care

This includes nursing care, pain relief and relief of other symptoms, and the offer of food and drink by mouth (perhaps with a spoon, straw or cup).

The code of practice produced by the British Medical Association states that patients can refuse life-prolonging medical treatment, but they cannot refuse basic care.

It can be difficult to think ahead to the future and personal values are very important for the process of advance planning. This is because end-of-life treatment decisions are made in the context of deeply held beliefs and personal views about what contributes to our quality of life. Two simple questions that may help your relative to think about this are:

- What makes your life worth living now?
- What would make your life not worth living in the future?

Your relative may want to ensure that the small things they value in everyday life continue if they become ill or incapacitated. This may include where they wish to be cared for or what information they would want to receive from their health professionals, such as whether they have a terminal illness or not. To elicit this information the person must consider those things that are important to them, which they want others to know about.

Some advance statements combine a record of personal values with a specific directive about treatment preferences. For example, if the only treatment for your relative is aggressive chemotherapy, radiotherapy or radical surgery, they may prefer to opt for palliative care which is to do with relieving symptoms of disease and in particular, supplying effective pain relief.

If your relative has made a living will, you should make sure you review what they have recorded periodically, to ensure their wishes have not changed.

Finding the Documents You Need For Your Loved One

Caring for a loved one involves many things and you may become a primary carer to your elderly relative as well as an advocate in legal circumstances. Whether you provide care yourself, co-ordinate or oversee carers or provide a watchful eye on your relative from a distance, you will need all the correct documentation in order to speak on their behalf or manage their affairs when they die.

It can be hectic managing more than one household. Anything you can do to make the tasks easier for yourself is good. When you need documentation, you want to know where it is so you can get your hands on it in a hurry. This simple matter of organising documents is more important than ever when you are responsible for a loved one. It brings peace of mind not only to your loved one, but also to you.

You will want to keep important documents stored safely inside a metal box or a safety deposit box. Be sure the documents are somewhere that is easy to find by you or other family members. Remember, you will be at your worst when the time comes to find and present these documents, so be sure you know where they are. Here is a short list of the documents you will want to locate.

Last Will and Testament

This is the documentation that tells you where your loved one wants their money, property, and goods to go when they pass on.

Medical information

In an emergency, you don't want to be fumbling around for a list of medication or the number for your relative's doctor. Keep a list of all of this information in a central location for easy reference.

List allergies, medications, and the length of time on medications. Keep this information updated.

Insurance information

Find the policies for all insurances including home, vehicle, health and life. Become familiar with policies so you know how much they are worth and what stipulations there are on pay outs. Many people miss out on having insurance pay for certain services for their loved one because they don't know where the information is. Many insurance companies now offer their policyholders an online version of the policy. Print that out and keep it safe.

Power of Attorney

This is important when your relative becomes incapacitated and needs someone to make decisions on their behalf. Even if a person is not incapacitated fully, you may have taken over paying bills or other simple money tasks.

Financial Information

You will need details of your relative's savings and investments and their income and outgoings in case you need to take over the management of their finances. List the name and account numbers of your relative's bank, building society, pension provider, saving accounts and details of any shares they may hold. Don't forget to include their national insurance number for correspondence about their state pension.

Protecting your loved one is all a part of taking care of them. Knowing where their important information and documents are located can help you to do that and save you a lot of stress at the same time. *Age UK* produce a free *Life Book*, to record and find important information that you may find useful. You can find their details in the helpful resources section.

End of life care

When a loved one becomes ill, it can be a distressing, frightening and lonely time, which can leave us with a sense of helplessness and loss of control. It is important that you share these worries and concerns with other family members or health professionals and find out what you can do to support your elderly relative on their final journey.

Your loved one may want to be cared for in their own home. Most people do, yet most die in hospital. I think this is a great shame and I will fiercely resist this happening to my own father. Your relative may already be in a care or nursing home like my mother. The same principle applies here. If they want to die in the place they have come to think of as their home then every effort should be made for this to happen. However the home will have the final say which is why it is important to ask about the home's policy on end-of-life care when your relative is choosing a home.

Richard's Story

When Richard's mother, Mabel, passed ninety and needed looking after, her son Richard shut up his home in Australia and came back to live with her. Richard was advised to put his mother in a nursing home soon after her ninety-fifth birthday, following a fall and her admission to hospital. Mabel was bed-ridden and needed care for all her basic needs, but Richard did not want his mother to die with strangers and wanted her home. He turned one of the rooms in her cottage into a ground floor bedroom and, with help, put a care package together. This included two carers attending his mother four times a day while he was at work and looking after her himself at night. Richard had a weekend break alternate months and a week off every six months to recharge his batteries, when carers moved in to look after Mabel. To everyone's surprise, his mother lived until she was over 100 and died peacefully at home with her family around her.

If your relative is in a care home when they make their final journey, they may need extra care. Palliative care should be available in a nursing home through registered nurses on the staff team and in a care home by bringing in district nurses or specialist nurses and equipment from your relative's GP. If your relative lives in a care home, they have the same rights as people living in their own home to specialist services available in the community.

If your relative has cancer or other life-limiting illness, such as motor neurone disease or a heart and lung condition, they may be able to access a hospice. A hospice is not just a building; it is a way of caring for people at home or as an in-patient. Hospices not only take care of people's physical needs, they consider their emotional, spiritual and social needs too. They also support families both during the illness and bereavement. The services offered will vary from hospice to hospice but are likely to include:

- Medical and nursing care
- Therapies, including physiotherapy and complimentary therapies
- Practical and financial advice
- Spiritual support
- Support in a person's own home
- Day care
- Respite care
- Residential support for treatment and pain management

When I was doing my social work training I spent a day at a hospice. Far from being depressing, it was a wonderfully positive experience. Patients were cared for in an individual and holistic way, could choose whatever they wanted to eat and drink and appeared pretty much pain free. One of the things I learned and have used when someone is ill or dying is to make ice cubes from pineapple juice. I crush them and put a small piece in the person's mouth to cool and refresh it. Try it yourself!

Dee's Story

Dee's mother, Maud, was diagnosed with bowel cancer at the age of eighty-five. Over the past six months her symptoms had become much worse and her doctors at the hospital wanted her to have another course of chemotherapy. Dee discussed this with her mother who was adamant that she did not want further treatment. Dee discussed her decision with Maud's GP who referred her to their local hospice. A week later, Maud was admitted to the hospice where they focused on keeping her comfortable and free of pain. Dee and her brother took it in turns to visit their mother every day. Maud died peacefully two weeks later and Dee and her brother were with her.

I have lost a number of elderly relatives, including both sets of grandparents, my parents-in-law, an aunt who I adored, other aunts and uncles as well as the man I was married to for more than thirty years. I have also had the privilege of sharing their final journey with many people when I worked in a hospital for older people (referred to, then, as a geriatric hospital) and managed care homes for older people. During this time I observed that for most people the final stage of life is very peaceful. Your relative may be in a coma, which can last for minutes or hours. Remember that people in comas can sense and hear sounds around them so continue to talk and touch them. This can be a really good time to tell your relative how much you love them, why you love them and talk about the happy memories they are leaving you with.

Practical arrangements to make after a death

The death of your relative can be a difficult time. You may be feeling a range of mixed emotions, including numbness, anger, grief and possibly even relief and guilt. In the short-term there will be practical decisions to make and things to do that will keep you busy. The following is a list of the things you will need to do. Try to keep a list of the people you need to contact, together with any notes, in a folder so that you can refer to them when you need to.

If your relative has died at home you need to contact their GP. If their death was expected they will give you a medical certificate showing the cause of death. You will also be given a formal notice stating that they have signed the medical certificate, telling you how to get the death registered. You will then need to contact the funeral directors. If your relative chose to be cremated you will need two doctors to sign separate medical certificates, but one of these can be completed any time before the cremation.

If your relative died in hospital, a medical certificate and formal notice will be issued by the hospital. The hospital will usually keep them in the mortuary until you have instructed funeral directors.

If the death was unexpected, or your relative's doctor has not seen them within the fourteen days before their death, the death will be reported to the police who will visit you. Don't worry about this, as it is usual practice. The police will then report the death to the coroner, who is a doctor or lawyer responsible for investigating unexpected deaths. He or she may call for a post-mortem. This is a medical examination of the body to find out more about the actual cause of death.

If your relative told you which funeral director they wanted before they died, you can contact them as soon as you have the medical certificate. Increasingly people like my parents are taking out a pre-paid funeral plan. If your relative has one of these, you need to find it straight away, as it will either state the funeral director to be used or give a number for you to ring to be told the information.

If your relative did not state the funeral directors they wanted, or did not take out a funeral plan, you will need to decide which one to use yourself and contact them. When you contact the funeral director they will want to know whether your relative is to be buried or cremated and arrange to collect and take them to their chapel of rest.

Registering a death

The death needs to be registered within five days (although this can be extended in certain circumstances) at the registry office of the area in which the death occurred. If this is a different area to the area in which you live, you can use your local office and they will forward the information on. Registration of a death is free of charge, however you will need several copies of the death certificate, which cost £3.50 at the time of writing. The registrar will need the following information:

- The medical certificate showing the cause of death.
- The full names of your relative (and any other names they once had).
- Their date and place of birth.
- The date and place of death.

- Their usual address.
- Their most recent occupation.
- Whether or not your relative was receiving a pension or other benefits.
- The name, occupation and date of birth of their spouse or civil partner.

If possible you should take your relative's medical card or NHS number and their birth and marriage certificate, if available.

The registrar will give you:
- A certificate for burial or cremation, which gives permission for the body to be buried or an application for cremation to be made.
- A certificate of registration of death. If your relative was receiving any benefits you should complete the form and send it to the Department of Work and Pensions.
- A death certificate if you want one. This will be needed for the will and any claims to pensions, savings etc. I suggest that you pay for several copies, as copies required later will be more expensive and photocopies are not accepted by some organisations.

Tell Us Once

Tell Us Once lets you report your relative's death to most government organisations in one go. You can also use the online service if you've already registered a death and have your 'Tell Us Once' reference number.

'Tell Us Once' is a relatively new service offered by most local authorities on behalf of the Department for Work and Pensions (DWP) to save time.

How to use Tell Us Once

Ask if your relative's local council's register offices offer the service when you're booking your appointment to register the birth or death. Not all do.

If they do, the registrar can help you use the service at your appointment, or you can do it yourself afterwards.

If they don't, you must register the birth or death and let relevant parts of government know about it yourself.

Using Tell Us Once will tell the right parts of government so they can:

- work out final payments of benefits for the person who's died (including the State Pension) and tax credits

- make arrangements for Income Tax, National Insurance and Council Tax.
- cancel the passport and/or driving licence of the person who's died (if you've provided this information)
- let local council services know so they can make arrangements about council housing and Blue Badge schemes
- make sure the person's name is removed from the electoral register (also known as the electoral roll)

It is essential to note that you must have registered the death and been given the unique Tell Us Once reference number before you can use the telephone or online service.

Arranging your relative's funeral

Once you are sure that the death does not have to be reported to the coroner, it is time to arrange the funeral. You will need to meet with your chosen Funeral Director either at their office or at home to discuss the date of the funeral and how you want it carried out. You will be asked about your relative, their life, occupation and character, any hymns or music you want played and whether you want flowers.

A basic funeral covers the following items:

- The Funeral Director's services.
- Provision of necessary staff.
- A coffin suitable for the purpose of cremation or burial.
- Transfer of the deceased from the place of death during normal working hours.
- Care of the deceased prior to the funeral.
- Provision of a hearse to the nearest crematorium or cemetery.
- Attend to all necessary paperwork and arrangements.

All work that is done outside normal working hours will mean extra costs. If these services are not all required, the bill should be reduced accordingly. There should be a price list for all the different types of coffin, casket, and services provided. The Funeral Director should provide a written estimate of all the costs involved, including the extra costs of embalming, flowers, cremation and cemetery fees and doctor's and clergy's fees.

Advising people about your relative's death

If your relative had a Christmas card list you can use this to let other relatives, friends, and neighbours know about your relative's death. You will also need to contact some or all of the following organisations:

- HM Revenue and Customs.
- DVLA.
- Office of the Public Guardian (if they had an Enduring or Lasting Power of Attorney).
- Personal or occupational pension providers.
- Mortgage provider, housing association or council housing office.
- Insurance companies.
- Bank and building society.
- Social Services (if your relative was getting any community care services or equipment).
- Utility companies.
- GP, dentist and anyone else providing medical care.
- The bereavement Register (to put a stop to post sent to people who have died).

Dealing with your relative's estate

Hopefully, your relative will have left a will giving details about what they want done with their property and other assets. It will also state who they wanted as executor to carry out their wishes. If you are the executor, in order to gain access to your relative's assets you will need to get a grant of probate from the Probate Registry. If your relative did not leave a will, but had money or property, you will need to make an application for legal authority to administer their estate to the Probate Registry. The Probate and Inheritance Tax Helpline can give you details of your local registry (see *Helpful Resources*) and can also give you general advice on getting probate.

Loss and bereavement

Whether anticipated or unexpected, losing a loved one can turn our world upside down and leave us feeling lost and overwhelmed. When caring for an elderly relative comes to an end after death, you can also feel an acute sense of loss, not only in respect of the person who has died. You may also face the loss of the relationships you built up with the professionals involved in your relative's care as well as the loss of your role and the occupation of looking after them. Suddenly you may find free time on your hands, which can make you feel confused and disorientated.

When I was managing care homes for older people, I was aware of the impact losing a loved one had on relatives and that this loss of role and the structure it offered left a big hole to fill. As a result I set up a visitors' group for residents who did not have anyone to visit and care for them. This offered relatives of people who had died a more flexible structure and the opportunity to continue to feel needed. It also improved the quality of life for residents who did not have visitors.

Losing someone we love can take us on a journey of bereavement, during which we face the powerful feelings of loss and grief. These feelings can be hard to make sense of and may be made worse because of other losses we have experienced during our life.

In addition to our own grief, we may also be left with a widowed parent or other elderly relative who may not want to carry on living without their partner. Their sadness and loneliness can affect us greatly at a time when we are struggling to come to terms with our own loss.

The many practical things we have to do when someone dies, such as registering the death and planning the funeral, keep us busy and to some extent, take our mind off our feelings. It is usually only after the funeral that we really begin grieving.

The time it takes to get over the grieving stage varies enormously and there are no hard and fast rules. Every journey will be unique. However, I can promise you that things will eventually get better. However, it is important that you take care of yourself during the grieving process and most importantly, talk through how you are feeling with family and friends or your GP. Having a nutritious diet, keeping active and giving yourself regular treats are equally important.

Allowing your feelings to come out can help you get used to your loss. Talking about the death and the person who died, dealing with the practicalities of your new situation, and trying to think of the present as well as the past can all help you become used to the reality of the death and get through some of the anguish you feel. You will slowly begin to find a way of living without the person alongside you, but very much with you in your thoughts and memories.

I will leave you with the wonderful words used at the Queen Mother's funeral and hope you find them as inspirational as I do.

Remember Me

Do not shed tears when I have gone, but smile instead because I have lived.

Do not shut your eyes and pray to God that I'll come back, but open your eyes and see all that I have left behind.

I know your heart will be empty because you cannot see me, but still I want you to be full of the love we shared.

You can turn your back on tomorrow and live only for yesterday, or you can be happy for tomorrow because of what happened between us yesterday.

You can remember me and grieve that I have gone, or you can cherish my memory and let it live on.

You can cry and lose yourself, become distraught and turn your back on the world or you can do what I want – smile, wipe away the tears, learn to love again and go on.

David Harkins

Points to remember

- Planning for end of life is important and needs to be done before your relative becomes too ill.
- A Living Will is a statement of a person's views about how they would like or not like to be treated if they are no longer able to make decisions.
- Creating a way to find important documents and information will save you time and frayed nerves.
- Losing a loved one can leave a gap that volunteering can fill and help you continue feeling needed.
- It is important that you take care of yourself during the grieving process.

Did you know?

Life expectancy in the United Kingdom has reached the highest level on record for both males and females.

ENDINGS

The end of the journey with my parents has arrived. Mum has settled into her new care home, as well as she will settle anywhere without my father. Staff there are kind, experienced and skilled in caring for people with dementia and I feel better knowing she is being well looked after by people who understand her condition.

Dad's life journey rapidly came to an end. His health had been deteriorating and days away from his 90th birthday, a milestone he desperately wanted to reach as no one in his large family had managed it, he lost his strength and became confined to bed. I moved in to care for him as he wanted to remain at home and I didn't want him to spend his last days in an impersonal and understaffed hospital ward with a high risk of infection. Neither did I want his life prolonged, as his quality of life had deteriorated badly. I discussed this with his GP, as I knew it is what Dad wanted, and kept the DNR (Do Not Resuscitate) form available in case it was needed.

In spite of knowing I was carrying out Dad's wishes, when I heard his worsening cough I wondered whether a trip to the hospital with antibiotics and IVs etc. would ease his discomfort. The thought was only fleeting and I was thankful we had discussed the matter before his health deteriorated.

Watching someone you love slipping away when there is nothing you can do about it is not easy. I felt as if I had stepped outside normal life and was suspended in some kind of time warp; I missed my home and my own bed. Dad had a worsening cough, spent most of his time sleeping and must have ached from being in bed so long. He also had a temperature caused by dehydration; not drinking enough causes a fever. I was glad he slept through the indignities to which he had to be subjected and I was startled by the realisation of how much like an infant Dad became. My heart ached when I reflected on the proud, upright and independent man he had been.

Dad became unable to move himself or follow the most basic instruction and moving and handling him required two people. His GP and the district nurse referred him to the NHS Continuing Healthcare End of Life Team. I told them I wanted to bring the care to Dad, not take him to the care. A hospital bed and turning sheet were ordered and we planned to move him into the lounge to give more space to care for him. I was told two carers would visit Dad four times a day. However, the bed and turning sheet were never delivered and only one agency carer arrived most of the time instead of two, which meant I had to be there to help them. When I was no longer able to give Dad morphine orally I requested a syringe driver: this never arrived either, and I seemed to spend most of my time on the phone chasing things and being answered by a machine. I received apologies from the district nurse, care provider and GP for their errors; and I had a sense of a care system for older people that is straining to cope. This can only get worse as numbers increase.

One of the biggest surprises to me was the contrasting experience of care provided by Social Services and the NHS. While I appreciated the amount and frequency of care Dad received from the NHS, I missed the control and flexibility I had from a Social Services personal budget. Care provided by the NHS appears to be used exclusively for personal care and not for helping carers with other tasks such as the huge amount of laundry, collecting prescriptions or giving me a break. I believe this is a good example of the need to integrate health and social care to deliver a more holistic service to people at the end of their life.

As the NHS took over responsibility for Dad's care, funding from Social Services stopped. I had to make his two Personal Assistants redundant, one of whom had been employed for over five years and had become more like a friend to Dad. My experience also made me aware of the difficulties family carers experience when their loved one cannot be left on their own and they have to cancel appointments and give up doing the things they want or need to do.

As Dad became unable to visit Mum at her care home, my brother brought her to see him at home. We were worried about how this would affect her and whether going back home would confuse her, but it went surprisingly well and played an important part in preparing her for her husband's death.

As each day passed and Dad's birthday came and went, I realised and began to accept that I was not in control. This was my father's journey. It was his choice to stay or go. I could walk beside him, but I could not change the outcome. It is hard to give up control, especially when death is the certain end, but it leaves us with an important life lesson: we do not have the control in life we think we have. We can only accept what life brings our way and choose instead to let it mould and shape us and provide depth and meaning to our character.

Dad passed away peacefully the day after his birthday, in his own home with his favourite music playing. I am so grateful I was able to spend his last days with him and hope I provided the comfort that I know Mum would have given had things turned out differently.

I miss him and my heart aches for what I have lost, but I know he is in a better place. As children we learn important life skills and values from our parents. As adults we can also learn a lot about ourselves if we open our heart and choose to share our parents' final journey with them.

ENDINGS

REFLECTIONS

- Caring for my parents has taken many twists and turns over the past few years. As their ability to function decreased, my involvement increased and it has sometimes felt as if I have taken one step forward and two steps back. The emotional roller coaster has taken its toll on us all.

- Becoming responsible for our parents is not something we plan for and does not always turn out as we anticipate. The wheels of change keep turning and my siblings and I can take comfort from the knowledge that we did, and are doing, the best we can for our parents. This is the most that anyone can do.

- Amongst the trials and tribulations I have experienced on my parents journey, I became even closer to my brother and sister and am truly grateful for their love and support as we shared our parents' final journey together.

- I have spent so much time running round in circles trying to do "the right thing" for my parents. No sooner did I get everything under control than something changed, but isn't that life? It's rather like a parcel. Every time we think we have packed it up a bit pops out and we have to reach for the *Sellotape* and stick it down again. I've come to realise that the most important thing we can do when caring for people we love is to learn to give up control over the things we cannot control.

- Another thing I learned along the way was that our parents' tastes could change, as they grow older. I found for example that my mother decided she would drink orange cordial whereas she used to hate it and doubled the sweeteners she had in her coffee. This made me realise that I could no longer assume things were the same as they had been at home.

- It is easy to become irritated by our relative's preoccupation with their health and frustration about their increasing dependence, but we need to remember that their world is shrinking to memories of the past and their current reality. They are beginning to close down, emotionally as well as physically, and have a need to look back, reflect upon and evaluate their life. That is why I asked my brother and sister to put together the picture life-story for Mum and why I encouraged Dad to talk about his travels with Mum and tell his war-time stories.

- When we are feeling tired or stressed it is easy to become frustrated. When caring for our relatives we need to practise patience, not only with our loved ones, but also with ourselves. Unfortunately I was at the back of the queue when patience was being handed out, so I have a lot of practice ahead!

- The saying "Yesterday has gone, tomorrow is yet to come, which is why today is called the present (a gift)" is so true. Today is all we have and we need to focus on the most valuable thing in each moment. Focusing on the quality of the time we spend with our elderly loved ones is so much more important than how much time we spend with them.

- We need to create space for ourselves if we are to continue to give to others. Driving ourselves into overload and becoming stressed is not good for us physically, mentally or emotionally and neither is it good for the loved ones we are trying to support. I learned this the hard way when I was taken ill on holiday with a pulmonary embolism. I blame it on having been too busy for physical exercise, going to the gym or out for a walk during the months leading up to leaving my job and going on holiday. My life was particularly stressful as I juggled a busy professional life and setting up a new business with caring for my elderly parents.

- What we need to do is find our own way of balancing our physical and emotional needs with the demands of our ageing parents and we need not do this alone. As well as friends and relatives there are carers support groups, on line forums and people we can talk to as well as getting practical help. There is lots of help out there so don't be afraid to ask for it.

- When my mother had to move into a care home and be separated from my father and her husband of sixty-four years, the emotional turmoil and guilt I felt were extraordinary and something I never expected. Having endorsed my mother's goal of keeping her at home with my father, I felt I had let her down. We therefore need to be careful not to make promises we may not be able to keep about care options that may be possible for our loved ones and take into account the impact they may have on the people closest to them.

- I will always be grateful to my mother's social worker for her support, not only for my mother, but also for me. It is just not possible to be objective with people we are very close to and we can get tangled up in our emotions, the strength of which should not be underestimated. It took the social worker's objectivity to cut through the baggage attached to Mum's relationship with my father, to get the right outcome for my mother and indirectly, my father. Having spent much of my life helping and supporting others, I also appreciated having professional support myself during this life-changing event for my parents.

The insight I gained from this will in turn help me support clients who are struggling to find the best care solution for their elderly loved ones without a social worker to help them.

- The care landscape is likely to change significantly over the coming years as Social Services departments and the NHS seek new ways to meet the demands of an ageing population. Having to do more with less will be their mantra and families will be expected to play an even bigger role in caring for their loved ones.

- It is therefore important that we become informed about what options are out there for older people and know what standards we can expect. Only then can we make the choices that underpin the person-centred approach that is at the heart of current health and social care reforms.

- I hope this book will help you with the choices you need to make and I wish you every success on the journey ahead with your own parents or elderly relative.

HELPFUL RESOURCES

Chapter 1 – The Care System and Assessment Matters

Age UK

Age UK provide information and advice for older people about a range of issues relating to older people, including: NHS services, assessment for community care services; NHS Continuing Healthcare; and NHS funded nursing care. Check them out at www.ageuk.org.uk or contact their Advice Line on 0800 169 6565.

Independent Age

A charity for older people that can advise on a range of issues and produces guides and fact sheets including guides about the Community Care system and Needs Assessment. You can find them at www.independentage.org. Alternatively, contact their Advice Line on 0845 262 1863 or their Order Line on 0207 241 8522.

NHS Choices

Provides clear extensive information about a range of things, including the NHS structure, Social Care

Assessments and NHS Continuing Healthcare. You can find them at www.nhs.uk.

Care Aware

A non-profit making information and advisory service, specialising in a range of issues relating to care for older people, including the care system and assessments. You can find them at www.careaware.co.uk or by calling their free Advice Line 0161 707 1107.

Care Directions

Provides a guide to care and the rights of older people. Includes information about Assessments and Social Care. You can find them at www.caredirections.co.uk.

Chapter 2 – Direct Payments and Personal Budgets

Age UK

Age UK has produced information on direct payments and personal budgets. You can find them at www.ageuk.org.uk.

NHS England

Provides information about Personal Health Budgets. You can find them at

www.personalhealthbudgets.england.nhs.uk.

Government website

Provides information about public services. See "Direct payments – arranging your own care and services" You will find it at www.gov.uk.

In Control

This organisation is one of the pioneers of Personal Budgets and produce lots of information you may find helpful. You can find them at www.in-control.org.uk.

Social Care Institute for Excellence (SCIE)

See SCIE report 40: keeping personal budgets personal at www.scie.org.uk/publications/reports/report40.

National Centre for Independent Living (NCIL)

NCIL is run by disabled people for disabled people and provides a wide range of publications relating to Direct Payments, Personal Budgets and arranging personal assistance. Check out their website at www.ncil.org.uk or Advice Line on 0845 026 4748.

Chapter 3 – Review and Complaint Matters

Patient Advice and Liaison Services (PALS)

Have been established to help people resolve problems, concerns and complaints about the NHS. Your can find your local PALS service by asking your GP surgery or local hospital. Alternatively you can find them on the NHS Choices website at www.nhs.uk. Alternatively you can phone NHS 111.

NHS Choices - Advocacy Services For Carers
Provide self-advocacy tips, information and advice about advocacy services with links to useful organisations. Check them out at www.nhs.uk.

SEAP (Support, empower, Advocate, Promote)
A free independent and confidential advocacy service that can help you make a complaint about any aspect of the NHS and social care. You can find them at www.seap.org.uk.

Age UK
Age UK, provides Information and advice about how to make a complaint about NHS and community care services. You can find their website at www.ageuk.org.uk or their Advice Line 0800 169 6565.

Independent Age
A charity for older people that can advise on a range of issues and produces guides and fact sheets including guides about how to complain when things go wrong. You can find them at www.independentage.org. Alternatively contact their Advice Line on 0845 262 1863.

Health & Care Professionals Council (HCPC)

The independent regulator for health and social care professionals. Hold a register of health and social care professionals. You can find them at www.hpc-org.uk or telephone 0845 300 6184.

Care Quality Commission

The independent regulator of health and social care services in England. Check them out at www.cqc.org.uk or telephone them at 0300 0616 161.

Advocacy

I have found advocacy services for older people to be patchy across the country but a good place to start is:

Older People's Advocacy Alliance (OPAAL)

OPAAL is the only national UK membership based organisation supporting, promoting and developing the provision of independent advocacy services for older people. You can find them at www.opaal.org.uk or telephone 01782 844 036.

Care Aware

A non-profit making information and advisory service, specialising in a range of issues relating to care for older people including an advocacy service. You can find them at www.careaware.co.uk or by calling their free Advice Line 0161 707 1107.

Chapter 4 – Hospital Discharge Matters

Age UK
Age UK provide information and advice for older people about a range of issues affecting older people including, going into hospital and hospital discharge arrangements Check out their website www.ageuk.org.uk or call their Advice Line 0800 169 6565.

Care Directions
Provides a guide to care and the rights of older people. Includes information about hospital discharge. You can find them at www.caredirections.co.uk.

Alzheimer's Society
Provides information about Alzheimer's and helpful information about discharge from hospital. Also an on line forum for people caring for someone with dementia. You can find them at the www.alzheimers.org.uk or look in your relative's phone book for their local office.

Carers UK
Offer a comprehensive range of information including discharge from hospital on their website www.carersuk.org or contact their free Carers Line 0808 808 777.

Chapter 5 – Care (Support) Planning Matters

NHS Choices
Provide information about a range of issues affecting older people including care (support) planning. Check them out at www.nhs.uk.

Independent Age
A charity for older people that can advise on a range of issues and produces guides and fact sheets including care (support) planning. You can find them at www.independentage.org. Alternatively contact their Advice Line on 0845 262 1863 or their Order Line on 0207 241 8522.

Helen Sanderson Associates
Provide a range of information and tools to help with care (support) planning. Check them out at www.helensandersonassociates.co.uk.

In Control
This site has lots of information including about care (support) planning. You can find them at www.in-control.org.uk.

Chapter 6 – Accommodation Matters

First Stop
Provides independent information and advice to older people and their families about housing and support options in later life. You can find out more at www.firststopadvice.org.uk or telephone 0800 377 7070.

Age UK
Age UK provide Information and advice for older people about a range of issues relating to older people including, accommodation. Check them out at www.ageuk.org.uk Alternatively contact their Advice Line on 0800 169 6565.

Citizens Advice Bureau (CAB)
A national network of free advice centres, including advice about national housing provision. Their website is www.citizensadvice.org.uk.

Homeshare International
You can find their website at www.homeshare.org or telephone 01865 699190.

Time finders
Offer a service created for older people who are moving from the family home into more convenient accommodation. Check them out at www.timefinders.org.uk.

Bridgefast

Offer a dedicated property related and home-move support service for older people. You can find them at www.bridgefast.co.uk or telephone 0333 4008121.

Chapter 7 – Environment and Equipment Matters

The Disabled Living Foundation

Provides a comprehensive range of information about different types of specialist equipment and have a number of detailed fact sheets on their website which you can find at www.dlf.org.uk or on their Helpline 0845 130 9177.

The Disability Equipment Register

Provides the largest single source guide of used second-hand disability equipment in the UK. You can find them at www.disabilityequipment.org.uk or telephone 0145 431 8818.

Turn2us

A charitable service, which helps people access grants and other help for adapting accommodation. Check them out at www.turn2us.org.uk or their free Helpline 0808 802 2000.

More Independent (MI)
Provide information about innovative products to help maintain independence. Check them out at www.moreindependent.co.uk.

Independent Age
A charity for older people that can advise on a range of issues. Also produces guides and fact sheets including guides about equipment. You can find them at www.independentage.org. Alternatively contact their Advice Line on 0845 262 1863 or their Order Line on 0207 241 8522.

NRS Healthcare
Provide products for better independence comfort and safety. You can find them at www.nrs.uk.co.uk or you can call them on 0845 485 7498.

Homecare Products
Offer a wide range of products to help people with a range of conditions from having a propensity for falling to a hearing or sight problem. For details of what is available visit www.homecare-products.co.uk or telephone 0843 224 1200.

Age UK
Age UK provide Information about equipment on their website www.ageuk.org.uk or on their Advice Line 0800 169 6565.

The Positive Ageing Company

Provides information about mobility and independent living equipment. Check them out at www.positiveageing.co.uk or you can telephone them on 0800 068 2582.

The Gadget Gateway

Provide information about assistive technology products and services to help maintain independence for longer. Check them out at www.gadgetgateway.org.uk.

Foundations

The national body for home improvement agencies in England. Home improvement agencies help older and vulnerable people maintain their independence by providing housing-related support. You can contact them at www.foundations.uk.com/home or telephone 0845 864 5210.

Trust Mark

Helps people find reliable, trustworthy trades people to make repairs and improvements to their homes. Check them out at www.trustmark.org.uk or telephone 0134 463 0804.

Insulation and draught proofing

Provides information about grants offered by local authorities. You can contact them on 0800 316 2808.

Red Cross

Offers a range of services including transport services and the loan of medical equipment. You can find their website at www.redcross.org.uk or telephone 0844 871 1111 to find your local branch.

Elderly Parents org

Uses concept of a virtual exhibition to showcase products and services for older people. Also provides information for adult children caring for elderly parents. Check them out at www.elderlyparents.org.uk.

Chapter 8 – Homecare Matters

The United Kingdom Homecare Association (UKHCA)

Provides contact details for homecare agencies that belong to them. All members comply with a code of practice. Also offers information about selecting a care service and a free leaflet called *Choosing care in your home*. You can find them at www.ukha.co.uk or telephone 0208 288 1551.

First Stop

Provides a home services directory, which aims to provide a wide range of services that help older people maintain their independence and quality of life at home. You can find out more at www.firststopadvice.org.uk or telephone 0800 377 7070.

Find Me Good Care
A website developed and managed by the Social Care Institute of Excellence (SCIE) to help people make choices about care and support. You can find them at www.findmegoodcare.co.uk.

The Care Quality Commission (CQC)
Offers a care directory of homecare agencies at www.cqc.org.uk.

Care At Home Today
Provide a home care and live-in care advice service and directory of home care services in the UK. Check them out at www.careathometoday.com.

Rest of their life
Aspire to offer a "one stop shop" to find and choose products and services for elderly loved ones. Check them out at www.restoftheirlife.com.

Independent Age
A charity for older people that can advise on a range of issues and produces guides and fact sheets including information about equipment. You can find them at www.independentage.org. Alternatively contact their Advice Line on 0845 262 1863 or their Order Line on 0207 241 8522.

Mailing Preference Service (MPS)

Free service funded by the direct (so called "junk') mail industry to enable people to have their names and home addresses removed from lists used by the industry. You can find their website at www.mpsonline.org.uk or telephone 0845 703 4599.

Telephone Preference Service (TPS)

A central opt-out register where people can register their wish not to receive unsolicited sales and marketing telephone calls. Check out their website at www.tpsonline.org.uk The TPS Registration Line is 0845 070 0707.

Women's Royal Voluntary Service (WRVS)

Your relative's local WRVS (see local phone book) may offer a choice of services including visiting schemes, shopping services, home-delivered meals, volunteer drivers and escort schemes. Check out their website at www.wrvs.org.uk or telephone 029 2073 9000.

Cinnamon Trust

A specialist charity for older people and their pets. Can help to re-home a pet if its owner is unable to take it to a care home. Their website is www.cinnamon.org.uk or telephone 0173 675 7900.

Chapter 9 – Residential Matters

The Relatives and Residents Association (RRA)

Provides support and information to older people and their relatives about going into care. You can check them out at www.relres.org or on their free Advice Line 020 7359 8136.

Find Me Good Care

A website developed and managed by the Social Care Institute of Excellence (SCIE) to help people make choices about care and support. You can find them at www.findmegoodcare.co.uk.

Compare Care Homes

Offers a free online care home comparison tool at www.comparecarehomes.com.

The Care Quality Commission (CQC)

Provides useful information about all registered care services, and inspection reports. They offer a directory of care homes can be found on The Care Quality Commission (CQC) website www.cqc.org.uk or telephone 0300 061 6161.

Age UK

Age UK provide Information and advice for older people about a range of issues relating to older people including, benefits and care fees advice. Check them out at www.ageuk.org.uk Alternatively contact their Advice Line on 0800 169 6565.

Independent Age

A charity for older people that can advise on a range of issues and produces guides and fact sheets including guides about what to look for in a care home. You can find them at www.independentage.org. Alternatively contact their Advice Line on 0845 262 1863 or their Order Line on 0207 241 8522.

Your Care Home

Offer a directory of care homes and related information. Check them out at www.yourcarehome.co.uk.

Chapter 10 – Residential Living Matters

First Stop

Provides a home services directory, which aims to provide a wide range of services that help older people maintain their independence and quality of life at home. You can find out more at www.firststopadvice.org.uk or telephone 0800 377 7070.

Relatives and Residents Association (RRA)

Supports care home residents and their relatives. You can find their website at www.relres.org.uk or telephone their Advice Line is 02073 598 136.

Age UK
Age Concern and Help the Aged are now Age UK. They provide Information and advice for older people about residential living on their website www.ageuk.org.uk or call the Advice Line on 0800 169 6565.

Independent Age
A charity for older people that can advise on a range of issues and produces guides and fact sheets about independent living. You can find them at www.independentage.org. Alternatively contact their Advice Line on 0845 262 1863 or their Order Line on 0207 241 8522.

Chapter 11 – Caring Matters

Carers UK
Offer a comprehensive range of information for carers on their website www.carersuk.org or contact their free Carers Line 0808 808 777.

Alzheimer's Society
Has information about caring for someone with dementia. You can find them on their website www.alzheimers.org.uk .

Carers Trust
A comprehensive site incorporating Crossroads who provide information, advice and support services to

carers. Check out their website at www.carers.org or telephone 0844 800 4361.

Carer's Allowance Unit

Provides information regarding Carer's Allowance, the main state benefit for carers, including eligibility and how to make a claim. You can find it on www.gov.uk/carers-allowance-unit or telephone 0177 289 9489.

NHS Carers Direct

Provides comprehensive care and advice for carers. You can find them at www.nhs.uk/carersdirect or you can telephone their confidential advice line 0808 802 0202 .

Silver Line

Supports older people by signposting them to services, offering a befriending service to combat loneliness and empowering those who may be suffering from abuse and neglect. Check them out at www.thesilverline.org.uk or telephone them on 0800 328 8888.

YECCO

A private social networking platform designed for and influenced by family carers offering a one-stop shop for connecting people, products and services. Check them out on www.yecco.com.

Vitalise

Provides holidays and respite care for people with severe disabilities with or without carers at five purpose-built centres in the UK. Also offers special Alzheimer's holidays for people with dementia and their carers, which are subsidised by the *Alzheimer's Society*. Check out their website at www.vitalise.org.uk or telephone 0845 345 1970.

Care Directions

Offer a guide to care and the rights of older people. You can find them at www.caredirections.co.uk.

Chapter 12 – Funding and Finance Matters

Independent Age

A charity for older people that can advise on a range of issues and produces guides and fact sheets about caring matters. You can find them at www.independentage.org. Alternatively contact their Advice Line on 0845 262 1863 or their Order Line on 0207 241 8522.

Government website

Online government services and information replacing Directgov and covering details of benefits and pensions and how to claim them. You can find them at www.gov.uk. (Use search bar to find what you are looking for.)

Society of Later Life Advisers (SOLLA)

A not-for-profit organisation that puts people in touch with accredited independent financial advice for older people. You can find their website at www.societyoflaterlifeadvisers.co.uk.

Care Fees Advice Agency

The Care Fees Advice Agency provides independent financial advice that specialises in helping people to find the best and most appropriate solution to the problem of funding long term care fees. Check them out at www.carefeesadvice.com or telephone 0800 078 7430.

Care Aware

A non-profit making public information, advisory and advocacy service specialising in elderly care funding advice in the UK. They also offer a helpful funding flow chart tool to identify potential eligibility for funding. Check out their website at www.careaware.co.uk they also have a free Helpline 0161 707 1107.

Department of Work and Pensions

Offer comprehensive information about the benefits you and your relative may be entitled to. You can find them at www.dwp.gov.uk. They also offer a free Benefits Enquiry Line 0800 882 200.

Turn2us
Offers a benefits checker, which can be used to find out whether your relative is entitled to benefits. They can be found at www.turn2us.org.uk or telephone 0808 802 200.

Age UK
Offer a Benefits Calculator, which you can access at www.ageuk.org.uk.

Carers Allowance Unit
Provides information regarding Carer's Allowance, the main state benefit for carers, including eligibility and how to make a claim. Check them out at www.direct.gov.uk or telephone 0845 608 4321.

The Pensions Service
Help with state pension eligibility claims and payments including pension credit. Check them out at www.gov.uk/contact-pension-service or you can give them a call on the following numbers: Making claims 0800 731 7898, General enquiries 0845 606 0265.

Care To Be Different
Provide practical information and specialist advice about care fees and NHS continuing healthcare. Also offer a 1 to 1 telephone advice service about

your specific situation in relation to NHS continuing healthcare. You can find them at www.caretobedifferent.co.uk.

The Money Advice Service
Offer clear, unbiased money advice, information and interactive money planners. You can find them at www.moneyadviceservice.org.uk.

Turn2us
A charitable service which helps people to access welfare benefits, grants and other help. Check them out at www.turn2us.org.uk or telephone 0808 802 2000.

Citizens Advice Service (CAB)
Offer an on-line guide about a range of issues including money and finance. You can find them at www.adviceguide.org.uk.

Bickers Insurance
Provide specialist home insurance to cover property while people are away in care homes on a temporary or long-term basis. Check them out at www.bickersinsurance.co.uk or telephone 0190 3791 340.

Chapter 13 – Legal Matters

Citizens Advice Bureau (CAB)
You can get free legal advice from the CAB and find your relative's local branch at www.citizensadvice.org.uk or look in their local phone book.

Government information
Provide information about public services all in one place including mental capacity and planning ahead and making decisions for someone else. You can find them at www.gov.uk (Use the search bar to find what you are looking for).

Patients Association
Produces information for patients about living wills. Telephone 0845 608 4455 or check out their website at www.patients-association.org.uk.

Solicitors for the Elderly
Solicitors for the Elderly are an independent national organisation of solicitors and barristers who are committed to providing a legal advice for older people and their families. You can find their website at www.solicitorsfortheelderly.com or you can ring them (mornings only) on 08700 670282.

Age UK
Provides information about making a will, lasting power of attorney and living wills. Also provides a

Wills Advice Service and helpful booklet, *Help with legal advice*. Check out their website at www.ageuk.org.uk or free Advice Line 08001 696565 or 08001 696565 for general enquiries.

Alzheimer's Society

Provides free information and guidance on preparing an advance decision. This information and a sample advance decision form can be downloaded from their website. www.alzheimers.org.uk and their Helpline on 0845 300 0336

Chapter 14 – Safeguarding Matters

Action on Elder Abuse

A specialist organisation with a focus exclusively on the issue of elder abuse. You can find their website at www.elderabuse.org.uk. They also provide a free Helpline on 080 8808 8141.

Age UK

Provide information about adult abuse and safeguarding. Check out their website at www.ageuk.org.uk. They also provide a free Advice Line 0800 169 6565 or 08001 696565 for general enquiries.

Solicitors for the Elderly

Produces a booklet for solicitors that gives details about financial abuse and action solicitors can take if they have concerns. Check out their website www.solicitorsfortheelderly.com.

Victim Support

Victim Support is an independent charity for victims of crime and has local offices across the country. You can find their website at www.victimsupport.org.uk or telephone their Victim Support Line 0845 3030 900 for support over the phone or to get details of your relative's local office.

Carers Trust

A comprehensive site which provides information, advice and support about legal issues. Check out their website at www.carers.org or telephone 0844 800 4361.

NHS Carers Direct

Provides comprehensive advice for about a range of issues including elder abuse. You can find them at www.nhs.uk/carersdirect or telephone their confidential advice line 0808 802 0202.

My Ageing Parent

A one-stop shop for advice on elderly care for ageing parents. You can find them at www.myageingparent.com.

Equality and Human Rights Commission (EHRC)

The EHRC has taken over the roles and functions of the Commission for Racial Equality and the Equalities Commission Check out their website at www.equalityhumanrights.com or telephone 0845 604 6610.

Trading Standards

If a person feels they have been charged an excessive amount of money for a service or been pressurised into buying something they did not want, Trading Standards may be able to help. You can find details about local offices on their website, www.tradingstandards.gov.uk Consumer Direct, a part of Trading Standards can be contacted on 0845 404 0506.

Chapter 15 – Family and Emotional Matters

Carers UK

Offers a forum and support for carers on their website www.carersuk.org and a free Carer's Line 0808 808 777.

NHS Carers Direct

Provides comprehensive care and advice for family carers. You can find them at www.nhs.uk/carersdirect or you can telephone their confidential advice line 0808 802 0202.

Alzheimer's Society

Provide an on line forum for people caring for someone with dementia. You can find them on their website, www.alzheimers.org.uk or look in your relative's phone book for their local office.

Elderly Parents org

Uses concept of a virtual exhibition to showcase products and services for older people. Also provides information for adult children caring for elderly parents. Check them out at www.elderlyparents.org.uk.

YECCO

A private social networking platform designed for and influenced by family carers offering a one-stop shop for connecting people, products and services. Check them out on www.yecco.com.

Depression Alliance

Helps people suffering from depression. It offers information and advice as well as a network of self-help groups and information leaflets. You can find their website at www.depressionalliance.org or telephone 0845 123 2320.

Citizens Advice Bureau (CAB)

Offer an on-line guide about a range of issues including family matters. You can find them at www.adviceguide.org.uk.

British Wheel of Yoga
Lists local yoga classes. You can find their website at www.bwy.org.uk or telephone 0152 930 6851

Keep Fit Association
Offer exercise and movement classes. Check them out at www.keepfit.org.uk or telephone 020 8692 9566.

Central Council of Physical Recreation
Offer advice on all sports. You can find them at www.ccpr.org.uk or telephone 020 7854 8500.

British Association for Counselling and Psychotherapy
Provide information about qualified counsellors and psychotherapists. Check out their website at www.bacp.co.uk or telephone 0870 443 5252.

National association for Mental Health (MIND)
Offers support to people in mental distress and their families. Check out their website at www.mind.org.uk and free Advice Line 020 8519 2122.

Sane
A mental health charity, that deals with mental illness including, anxiety and depression. Telephone Saneline 0845 767 8000.

The Samaritans
Offers a 24-hour Helpline for those in distress on 0845 790 9090.

Chapter 16 – Dementia Matters

Alzheimer's Society

Provides comprehensive information about Alzheimer's and other dementias. Also an on line forum for people caring for someone with dementia. You can find them at the www.alzheimers.org.uk or look in your relative's phone book for their local office.

Dementia UK

Their mission is to improve the quality of life for people affected by dementia and also to promote and develop Admiral Nursing. Admiral Nursing DIRECT is a national helpline and email service, provided by experienced Admiral Nurses for family, people with dementia and those worried about their memory. It gives practical advice and emotional support to anyone affected by dementia. Call them on 0845 257 9406 or email direct@dementiauk.org.

Dementia Care Matters

A national organisation that focuses on initiatives that focuses on Mattering in Dementia Care. Check them out at www.dementiacarematters.com.

Contented Dementia Trust

The Contented Dementia Trust is a small charity that aims to promote well-being for people living with dementia through teaching and use of the

SPECAL method. You can find them at www.contendeddementiatrust.org.

Dementia Web
Provide information prescriptions, handy guides, hints & tips for people living with dementia. You can find them at www.dementiaweb.org They also offer a 24 hour dementia helpline on 0845 120 4048.

Alzheimer's Research
The UK's leading dementia research charity, specialising in finding prevention, causes, treatments and a cure for dementia. Check them out at www.alzheimersresearchuk.org.

Dementia Challengers
Signpost Carers to on-line information and resources for people living with and affected by dementia. Check them out at www.dementiachallengers.com.

at dementia
Information on assistive technology for people living with dementia www.atdementia.org.uk.

Just Checking
Offer a simple system that helps people to live independently. Check them out at www.justchecking.co.uk or telephone 01564 785 100.

Lily pins

Lily Pins Ltd is the only company in the UK providing CRB checked, Dementia Trained, hairdressers, beauticians and chiropodists exclusively to residential and nursing homes and care centres. You can find them at www.lilypins.co.uk.

Active Minds

Provide a range of activity products for people living with dementia. You can find them at www.active-minds.co.uk.

2 find-me

A tailored safety system in a watch that is not limited to the person's home. Check it out at www.2findme.co.uk.

Chapter 17 – End of Life Matters

Bereavement Advice Centre

Provide support and advice to people on what they need to do after death. You can find them at www.bereavementadvice.org or telephone 0800 634 9494.

Cruse Bereavement Care

Helps people understand their grief and cope with loss. As well as counselling and support it offers information and advice. Check out their website www.cruse.org.uk.

The Bereavement Register

A service designed to remove the names and addresses of people who have died from databases and mailing files. You can register by accessing their website at www.the-bereavement-register.com/uk or telephone 0870 600 7222.

Hospice Information Service

Check out their website at www.hospiceinformation.info or telephone 0207 520 8222.

Marie Curie Cancer Care

For information on cancer care and Marie Curie nurses. Check out www.mariecurie.org.uk or telephone 0800 716 146.

Macmillan Cancer Line

For information on cancer care and Macmillan nurses, check out www.macmillan.org.uk or telephone 0808 808 0000.

Probate and Inheritance Tax Helpline

Telephone 0845 302 0900.

Probate Registry Helpline

Telephone 0845 3020 900.

Age UK

Provide information about all aspects of end of life planning and care as well as what to do when someone dies. Check out their website at www.ageuk.org.uk, their free Advice Line 0800 106 96565 or look in your relative's phone book for their local office.

The Well Planned Funeral
Offer a range of resources to help people plan their funeral.
Check them out at www.thewellplannedfuneral.com.

Dignity in Dying
Dignity in Dying campaigns for greater choice, control & access to services at the end of life. You can find them at www.dignityindying.org.uk or telephone 0207 479 7730.

Compassion in Dying
Provides information and resources to inform end of life choices.
Check them out at www.compassionindying.org.uk.

Pro Choice Living Wills
Offers a Living Will that has been put together by leading lawyers, doctors and nurses. Contact their website at www.livingwill.org.uk or telephone 0870 777 7868.

The Natural Death Centre
Provides information about woodland burials, cardboard coffins, living wills, funeral wishes form and do-it-yourself funerals. You can find their

website at www.naturaldeath.org.uk or their Helpline on 0196 271 2690.

Life Box

Offer a Life Box to store important information required by close family and executor when a person dies. Also stores personal details, life story, photographs and achievements etc. to give future generations accurate insight into the person's life. You can find them at www.mylastsong.com.

National Association of Widows

Information and support for those who have been widowed. Provides a supportive social life and friendship network via local branches. Check them out at www.nawidows.org.uk or telephone 0845 838 2261.

GLOSSARY

Advocate. An advocate is a person who speaks on behalf of another, or helps them speak up for themselves.

Assessment of need. The process to clearly identify what health or social care needs a person may have. It is completed by an assessor (such as a social worker or nurse) in partnership with the individual, their relatives or representatives.

Broker/Brokerage. Someone who helps individuals choose and access the support they need to be as independent as possible. Brokerage is the service offered by a broker.

Care home. A home registered with the Care Quality Commission (CQC) providing personal support or nursing as well as living accommodation.

Carer. A person providing care and support who is not employed by an agency or organisation. A carer is often a relative or friend supporting someone at home who is frail, ill or requiring support.

Community Care. Support provided to assist people in their day-to-day living.

Consent. The legal agreement to a choice or action made freely by an individual without pressure.

Direct payment. Payments made to an individual following a community care assessment in lieu of services.

Eligibility criteria. Provide the framework used to determine who is eligible for social care services from their local authority.

Financial assessment. A financial assessment is a means to identify whether an individual can make a contribution towards their care. Depending on an individual's financial circumstances, they may be asked to make a financial contribution towards the cost of their care and support.

Homecare. Support services provided to an individual in their own home by a care worker paid to provide care as part of their employment. Home care is also known as domiciliary care/support.

Local authority. Local authorities are democratically elected local bodies with responsibility for discharging a range of functions as set out in local government legislation.

Long-term care. Care and support that a person requires over a long period of time. This can be provided in an individual's home, care home or nursing home to assist people with their day-to-day living.

Personal assistant. A person employed to provide someone with social care and support in a way that is right for them. They can be employed directly by the individual or they can be arranged through an agency.

Personal budget. Social care funds allocated to an individual who is eligible for funding from Social

Services that can be used to meet their assessed eligible needs in a way that is right for them.

Personal health budget. A personal health budget is similar to a personal budget but applicable to health care. Patients with a personal health budget are able to take control over the way in which the budget available to them is spent. They can choose the support services they want in a way that is most appropriate to them.

Personalisation. Refers to the way in which services are tailored to the needs and preferences of people who use services and their carers.

Reablement. A short-term service, usually up to six weeks, for people who need support to live in their homes independently.

Rehabilitation. A process involving a number of different professionals which supports an individual to function physically, socially and psychologically.

Respite. When a carer is assessed as needing a break from caring, respite provides carers with a temporary break. This may be for very short periods of a few hours, or for longer periods of time.

Review. A review refers to the re-assessment of people's needs and circumstances.

Safeguarding. A process of ensuring that vulnerable people are protected from being abused neglected or exploited.

Support Plan. A document setting out how an individual's care and support needs are to be met. A support plan identifies what type of support an individual requires to meet their eligible need/s.

Telecare. A combination of equipment, monitoring and response designed to help individuals remain independent. It includes basic community alarm services able to respond in an emergency and provide regular contact by telephone as well as sensors, which detect things such as falls, flood, fire or gas and trigger a warning to a response centre or family member/carer. Telecare can also provide security by protecting against bogus callers, domestic abuse and burglary.

ABOUT THE AUTHOR

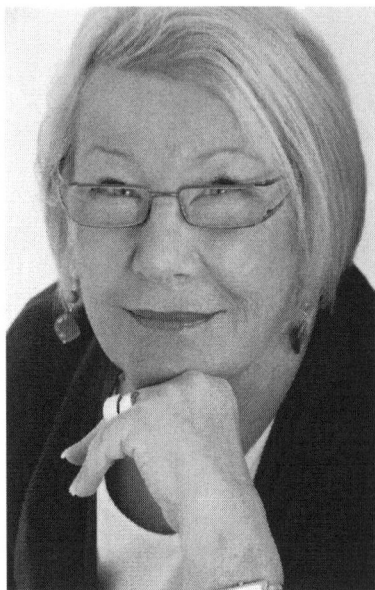

Chris Moon-Willems is regarded as a respected voice for family carers based on her extensive experience in social care and the NHS combined with personal experience of caring for her elderly parents. She became one of the pioneers of personal budgets, and their influence on personalisation, at a national and local level in social care and the NHS.

Chris gained important insight into personalisation when her parents were among the first older people in the country to be given a personal budget to buy their own services. She appeared on Breakfast TV to tell the story of their journey from having traditional services to personalised care and support and was interviewed on national radio stations.

As founder and owner of her elderly care consultancy, Relative Matters, Chris has created a dynamic business devoted to serving the needs of relatives and their ageing loved ones. What started out as a simple desire to share the story of her journey with her elderly parents has escalated into this book and her new business.

Chris is a qualified and registered social work professional, Master NLP Practitioner and a life coach. She has a passion and skill for helping older people and their families to think outside the box for ways to meet their needs and circumstances in creative ways that respect the individual and give value for money.

Chris can be contacted at chris@relativematters.org

9385019R00193

Printed in Great Britain
by Amazon.co.uk, Ltd.,
Marston Gate.